D1570156

# TIME
# MANAGEMENT
## FOR HEALTH CARE PROFESSIONALS

Steven H. Appelbaum and Walter F. Rohrs

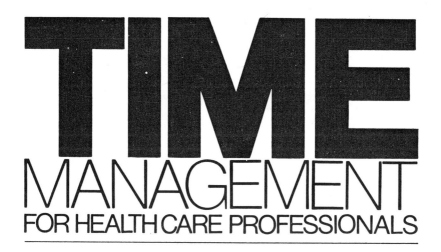

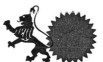

AN ASPEN PUBLICATION®
Aspen Systems Corporation
Rockville, Maryland
London
1981

Library of Congress Cataloging in Publication Data

Appelbaum, Steven H.
Time management for health care professionals.

Includes bibliographies and index.
1. Health services administrators — Time management.
2. Time management.   I. Rohrs, Walter F.
II. Title.
RA971.A8            362.1'068'5            81-3512
ISBN: 0-89443-378-4                              AACR2

Copyright © 1981 Aspen Systems Corporation

Library of Congress Catalog Card Number: 81-3512
ISBN: 0-89443-378-4

*Printed in the United States of America*

2 3 4 5

To *Barbara, Jill, Wendy, and Geoffrey Appelbaum*
and
*Helen Rohrs*

# Table of Contents

# Preface

Time is all we have. It is a common denominator and a scarce resource. It is cherished and respected, cannot be stored or recycled, is the fourth dimension, and is priceless. It is the criterion by which we measure a manager's accomplishments and effectiveness and eventually the achievements of his life. However, not every manager uses this resource to its best advantage. This may be due to contingencies and constraints over which he has no control, or it may be a result of a basic lack of knowledge and skills in managing resources and time.

Health care administrators are pressured, their work fragmented, and their future uncertain. They need to plan, to look ahead, and to be future oriented in order to adapt and cope with anxieties and demands within a climate of discontinuity. The health care environment is occupied with the juggling of productivity and quality care, which impacts upon the proper utilization of time. The management of time is one process by which administrators can achieve organizational goals and personal agendas that will enable them to be more effective in their personal and professional lives.

Theory and practice are not congruent, however. In North America, output per worker is increasing with mechanization and technology and the work week is shorter, but the hours needed by chief administrators have increased at a spiralling rate. Something is wrong and in need of managing. Managers have difficulties ascertaining the differences between what is urgent and what is important. Urgency engulfs the manager and yet the seemingly most urgent task is rarely the most important. What is missing is the concept of priorities. Peter Drucker has made a crucial point regarding this dilemma: Time is the scarcest resource and unless it is managed, nothing else can be managed. There is no single method to

---

*Note:* This book follows the standard practice of using a ''masculine'' pronoun wherever the pronoun refers to both males and females. ''Feminine'' pronouns appear only where antecedents are exclusively female.

use in managing time. A combination of the essential elements covered in this text is the formula recommended by the authors to effectively control this resource.

This book will deal with the following factors within the process of effective time management: planning, delegation, productivity, managerial roles, objectives-priorities, time traps, and stress. In addition to the theory and practice that have been interwoven within each chapter, the final chapter presents actual interviews with three executive directors of major metropolitan hospitals to discover how they effectively manage their time.

The authors wish to acknowledge the assistance given in this undertaking by Diane Tremaine and Derek Frost, research assistants at Concordia University, Montreal.

This book has been written for those health care managers and graduate students who need a model of effective time management. Management is both an art and a science. The synthesis of these aspects is the goal of this book.

*Steven H. Appelbaum, Ph.D.*
*Walter F. Rohrs, Ph.D.*

# Chapter 1

# The Management of Time

**TIME MANAGEMENT HIGHLIGHTS**

1. Individuals who keep up with change and manage to adapt well seem to have a more complete sense of what lies ahead. Planning for the future is subject to continued revision, which necessitates a contingency for flexibility. Formal planning must be future oriented, enabling those administrators in control to be future conscious. This can neutralize the trauma of time.

2. The importance of time management lies in the fact that many people have too many tasks they need to do but not enough time for the things they want to do and this often creates stress. Time management is a process by which you are more likely to attain or fulfill a need or desire.

3. In North America, the output per worker is increasing with mechanization and computerization; the work week is becoming shorter, and fringe benefits are multiplying, while the hours that are needed by the chief administrator are increasing at a spiralling rate. Long hours are not always conducive to accomplishment, although unfortunately, accomplishment and hours have been perceived as being synonymous.

4. Most of a manager's day is unstructured, with various blocks of discretionary time and an equal variety of discretionary tasks. The matching of tasks and time is one of the most important functions of the manager. Those who use time well focus on results and not tasks and activities.

5. Managers must not only be efficient but must be results oriented. There is a vast difference between being busy and being productive. The effort expended should be merely a means and not an end in

itself. The basis for an individual's value to an organization is in productive time rather than total elapsed working time.
6. Before a manager attempts to manage others, he must understand what he does in his job, his role, and with his time. Managers can save time by delegating more, saying no, working faster, setting priorities, and filtering interruptions that cut into efficiency.

## TIME?

The management of time is one of the most significant problems while at the same time a valued asset for managers of health care organizations. Probably more than many of us realize, time is both a scarce and valuable resource. While it is constantly and continuously available, it cannot be recycled, restored, or deposited in a bank to be withdrawn for future use. In addition, the limits of human endurance and capacity impose strong constraints on the extent and degree of intensity of its use. At some point, depending on individual differences, commitment of additional time appears to result only in progressively lower levels of output and, often concurrently, at a cost of even a greater expenditure of effort. As such, this important resource must be conserved, allocated, and used effectively, efficiently, and judiciously.

Abraham Maslow, the eminent psychologist, began one of his books by reproducing a photograph of small children laughing and smiling. Directly below was a picture of haggard adults with weary, drawn expressions. Captioning the two pictures were two words: "What happened?"

What happened was documented by a study at the California Institute of Technology (Newman, 1977, p. 8). Eleven hundred professionals and managers were surveyed about how well they managed their professional and personal time. Five out of six reported that they felt defeated by the age of 35 because they realized they had failed to fulfill their lives in two major ways: Some of their lifetime goals had proved unrealistic and, therefore, unattainable, and worse yet, they had been ineffective in managing those goals that were realistic. What can be done through time management to make life more fruitful?

The management of time is as much a personal dilemma as it is an organizational problem. The issue is now being addressed in various forms of research and popular literature intended to illuminate the problem and, hopefully, its ramifications and/or consequences.

Our free time, while technically increasing, is in fact decreasing. Among the active middle class, there is a sense of time rushing by; we feel frazzled, hectic, harried. We are experiencing a famine of time.

Part of this comes from having too many things to deal with, and it pains us. The painful effect of not having enough time for important things is threefold: (1) We do not get the pleasure we expect and require, resulting in chronic frustration, a lack of (or a souring of) our satisfaction. (2) We are violating a cultural imperative. In our culture, a person should spend sufficient time on children, family, sex, food, self-improvement, upkeep of homes and possessions; the reality (we don't have time for it) pales before it should, and guilty feelings result. (3) The conviction that we aren't spending the ''approved'' allotment of time on these activities makes us even more resolved to compress more into less time, escalating us into yet more harried and frantic behavior.

We've inherited a linear, segmented, future-oriented image of time, as well as a work time/free time split. Work time we make the best of, endure, or surrender to; it is generally not our own to do with as we please, and we are under compulsion to be productive for someone else. Our free time is what's left over, but every day we're pressed from another side to turn our free time into pseudowork time.

The ''efficiency'' methods used to run a business may work for business, but they fail miserably when used to eke satisfaction out of personal life. Applying such principles as ''time is money'' to your home life wreaks havoc. Unhappiness, dissatisfaction, feelings of being frazzled and harried and of never accomplishing anything worthwhile—all these result (Fanning & Fanning, 1979, pp. 151-152).

Our preoccupation with time and time consumption has been a traumatic event in our lives. In a column entitled ''Time's flying—and costs are soaring,'' appearing in the *Montreal Gazette,* Don Sellar gave the following facts and observations:

WASHINGTON—Time flies—it always has. But in the U.S. it seems to fly even faster than it once did.

It took 37 months for the General Dynamics-built F-16 jet fighter to go from first test flight to delivery of the 100th production model.

But it will take 61 months for the new McDonnell Douglas F-18, the new fighter that Canada recently bought, to reach the same milestone—if U.S. President Jimmy Carter doesn't cancel the program first.

That's a difference of two and a half years.

Back in 1931, the first tenant moved into the newly-completed Empire State Building in New York only 14 months after the ground-breaking.

But in Washington, the Phillip Hart Senate Office Building—a much less ambitious project—has a seven-to-10-year construction timetable that began in 1976.

At an informal backyard cookout, an American medical researcher from the world-renowned National Institutes of Health (NIH) bemoans all ''the terrible inertia.''

He says time-consuming delays in NIH plant expansion make it more attractive to give grants to outside researchers who work in independent labs.

To test a new drug, the U.S. Food and Drug Administration errs on the side of caution. Sometimes, 5,000 or even 10,000 mice are used in experiments that last nine months.

*Mice expensive*

The cost of keeping a single laboratory mouse fed, watered and housed for one day has reached the $1 plateau, so it's not too difficult to estimate the added costs involved when a test involving 10,000 mice is prolonged.

Not only does The Great American Delay cost money, but it's also credited with undermining the country's defense system, hurting productivity, fueling inflation and generally fouling things up.

Recently, Business Week magazine, in a lengthy discourse on the slow agony of U.S. re-armament, noted that some F-15 fighter planes will be built without engines until midway through 1981.

The problem? Strikes at two bearing and forging manufacturers have left Pratt & Whitney, the engine builder, short of engine parts.

Meanwhile, the U.S. Army and the Chrysler Corporation are engaged in a time-consuming exercise to produce the new Abrams XM1 tank, which is central to U.S. and NATO defense strategy for Europe.

Having spent eight years on this project, the Army and Chrysler— both repeatedly claiming the tank's technical problems have been solved—last spring made an announcement about production.

It has been delayed from June, 1983 until February, 1986. This will stretch the timetable for 7,058 Chrysler-built tanks to a full decade, if of course, Chrysler survives.

It's easy to finger the villains of delay—governments, regulators, courts, interest groups, business and labor.

*Everyone's a villain*

Trouble is, that's nearly everyone.

In an engaging essay on the problem, Pat Choate, a visiting fellow here at the Academy for Contemporary Problems, warns:

"If we are serious about reversing the decline in American productivity, the rise in unemployment, persistently high inflation and the deterioration of our military position in the world, we can start by eliminating The Great American Delay. There's little time to lose."

Choate believes it would take hundreds, even thousands of time-reducing actions by government to meet the challenge. Broad brush strokes wouldn't work, he says, because they would dismantle cherished democratic freedoms.

It's no gentle irony that the U.S.—the source of near-clichés such as "good old-fashioned American know-how"—should find itself grappling for solutions to such a basic problem.

It seems a long time ago that John F. Kennedy set a deadline of 10 years for an American to walk on the moon, a deadline that was met with several months to spare.

It appears that we need a measuring device to compare highly diverse processes. This device is time, which is often viewed as the interval during which most events happen. Events and situations are often difficult to measure and systematize for reliability, since they involve a separate dimension that is frequently overlooked because it cuts across all others. This is duration—the span of time over which a situation occurs. Two situations alike in all other respects are not the same at all if one lasts longer than another. Time enters into the mix in a crucial way, changing the meaning or content of situations. Just as the funeral march played at too high a speed becomes a merry tinkle of sounds, so a situation that is dragged out has a distinctly different flavor or meaning than one that strikes us in staccato fashion, erupting suddenly and subsiding as quickly (Toffler, 1972, p. 33).

The manner in which we respond to time often creates problems when we try to utilize it to achieve objectives. There may be a biological basis for differences in subjective response to time. "With advancing age," writes psychologist John Cohen (1964) of the University of Manchester, "the calendar years seem progressively to shrink. In retrospect every year seems shorter than the year just completed, possibly as a result of the gradual slowing down of metabolic processes." In relation to the slowdown of their own biological rhythms, the world would appear to be moving faster to older people, even if it were not (Toffler, 1972, p. 40).

The rapid pace that often appears uncontrollable has a greatly needed component of adaptation and coping to neutralize the counterproductive effects of this most complex, yet fascinating phenomenon. Toffler (1972, p. 419) describes this factor of anticipatory management:

This conditioned ability to look ahead plays a key role in adaptation. Indeed, one of the hidden clues to successful coping may well lie in the individual's sense of the future. People among us who keep up with change, who manage to adapt well, seem to have a richer, better developed sense of what lies ahead than those who cope poorly.

Anticipating the future has become a habit with them. The chess player who anticipates the moves of his opponent, the executive who thinks in long range terms, the student who takes a quick glance at the table of contents before starting to read page one, all seem to fare better.

Toffler further expands upon this factor:

The individual's sense of the future plays so critical a part in his ability to cope. The faster the pace of life, the more rapidly the present environment slips away from us, the more rapidly future potentialities turn into present reality. As the environment churns faster, we are not only pressured to devote more mental resources to thinking about the future, but to extend our time horizon—to probe further and further ahead (p. 420).

Planning for the future is subject to continual revision, necessitating a contingency for flexibility. Formal planning must be future oriented, which will ultimately make those administrators in control future conscious and help to neutralize the trauma they often experience with time.

Another article appearing in the *Montreal Gazette* entitled "Always late for work? You're slave of clock" also focused upon the trauma of time but yielded some solutions:

LONDON, Ont. (CP)—Some people are always late.

Psychologist Susan Shnidman says the person who is late for work arrives under stress and in an emotional mess. It's the late person, not the punctual one, who is really the slave of the clock, she says.

Shnidman, of Lexington, Mass., says chronic lateness may occur for a variety of reasons.

Some people want attention or want to express dissatisfaction with the task they are scheduled to do. At work, lateness can stem from a basic dislike for the job—an unwillingness to give up "your" time for "theirs."

Others are perfectionists and can't start another task until the one at hand is completed to the last detail. Some schedule too much for one day and end up going from pillar to post, perpetually one step behind in their own self-imposed regimen.

Whatever the cause, the late people inevitably bear the label among their friends and co-workers. They need to learn the day-to-day living skill of how to manage their time.

The first step in curing chronic tardiness, as in any problem-solving venture, is to realize that one exists.

For several days, keep a brief diary of what you do each day. See how long it takes to get out of bed, how long before anything is accomplished.

Ask yourself honest questions about your morning routine. Do you dally over what to wear? Do you fail to include the walk to the bus in your estimate of how long it will take to get to your destination? Do you know what you would like to do so that you have some direction, or do you drift?

Planning the day's activities is the key, especially if tasks are put in some order of importance. They can be labelled "Must do this," "Would like to get this done" and "Not necessary until later in the day."

Shnidman says there are several ways to improve time habits, and one of the best ways is to emphasize the positive consequences of arriving a little early (August 2, 1980).

Time management is one process by which managers and individuals can achieve the goals that will enable them to be effective in their lives and positions. Within this process there are several essential phases, whose purpose is to identify needs and wants in terms of importance and match them with the time and resources available. The goals needed to perform or achieve are prescribed by the organization, while those that the managers want to perform or achieve are imposed by their personal value system or related to their long-term career objective. The real importance of time management lies in the fact that many people have too many tasks they need to do, but not enough time for the things they want to do, which creates stress. If you are not able to attain or fulfill a need or desire, then according to definition you are experiencing tension and eventually stress. Time management is a process by which you are more likely to attain or fulfill a need or desire (Schuler, 1979, p. 852).

Preoccupations and frustrations involved with accomplishing the tasks of their job within a prescribed time slot do not permit managers to enjoy the intricacies of their role and maintain personal relationships that are supportive and satisfying and that could help to resolve some of the personality conflicts which are inherent in the overall symptoms of stress that they experience. It is interesting to note that in North America the output per worker is increasing with mechanization and computerization, the work week is shorter, and fringe benefits are multiplying, while the hours that are needed by the chief administrators of major organizations have increased at a spiralling rate.

## MANAGING THE RESOURCE

It is not uncommon for managers to work a 60 to 70 hour week while at the same time their employees are putting in a week approximately one-half of that time. Long hours for health care administrators are not always conducive to accomplishment since, unfortunately, accomplishment and hours have been perceived as being synonymous.

Management, it has been said, is a series of interruptions interrupted by other interruptions. Finding enough time to do all the routine things that must be done in addition to putting out the daily "fires" can be both difficult and demanding. Managers often feel that they need to work twice as fast as before just to stay where they are. Increasingly, return on invested time is as important as return on invested money. The amount of time it takes to complete a project or perform an assignment becomes a primary criterion in evaluating its success or failure.

Since most of a manager's day is unstructured—with various blocks of discretionary time and an equal variety of discretionary tasks—matching tasks and time can be one of the most important functions performed.

Those who use time wisely focus on results and not on tasks or activities. They learn to structure their environment so that it is conducive to concentration. They learn to distinguish between all the pressing and popular demands on their time and those things that actually require attention. Time is a valuable resource. Unless it is managed well, nothing else can be (Hill, 1976, pp. 26-27).

Many interesting statements have been made about time and time management. Benjamin Franklin once said, "To love life is to love time, since time is the stuff of which life is made." Individuals' personal characteristics and values greatly influence how they use time. More important, efficient management of time is based on respect for it (Scott, 1978, p. 56).

In *The Effective Executive,* Peter Drucker expresses concern as to how executives utilize their time and strongly urges the adoption of "systematic time management" as a diagnostic technique for obtaining a better allocation of this "totally irreplaceable and scarcest resource" (1967, p. 26).

Drucker suggests the following four steps (pp. 26-28):

1. Find out how you actually use your time.
2. Determine what doesn't have to be done and discontinue doing those things.
3. Delegate work to others who are equally or better qualified than you are.
4. Stop wasting other people's time.

The notion of the importance of time, however, is not merely restricted to the business world and the executives of profit-oriented enterprises. It is certainly at least equally significant to all health care professionals as they perform a wide range of duties in the various functions and levels of health care organizations. The need to manage time pervades all facets and activities of this increasingly important and sophisticated field.

In 1968, at a conference of 22 hospital administrators, attention was directed to time use, and a summary report of that meeting included these statements (Adams & Ponthieu, 1969, p. 46):

> One of the most challenging problems, it seems, that many hospital administrators face today is how to manage their time effectively. They do waste a large amount of their time and often the time of others. In fact they do it everyday.
>
> Not all of this time waste is their own fault. The routine demands of the organization, of professionals and of staff personnel eat away at the available time. Yet, they waste enough through their own misuse and mismanagement to hamper their productivity seriously.

In discussing a time study of five administrative staff members at one large hospital, Connors and Hutts (1967, p. 46) make these observations:

> . . . it behooves administrators in the health sectors of management to focus attention on the problem by studying what managers now do. . . . Because hospitals have purposes and goals that defy easy measurement of achievement, so also does the management of health institutions have difficulty in measuring its effectiveness and relating its functioning to the achievement of the goals of the institution. In the absence of precise standards of management activity and tested measures of the effectiveness of the activity, managers must look to what they are doing now in order to gain an understanding of what actually is happening in their institutions with the available administrative talent. . . . The paucity of management practice as it exists, on an empirical basis, is a first step in studying the endeavors that are described glibly as management and administration.

Management is constantly juggling the urgent and the important. One cannot ignore long-term consequences for the pressures of the moment. Managers must determine the difference between the urgent and the important. Urgency engulfs the supervisor, and yet the most urgent task is rarely the most important.

Supervisors or managers must not only be efficient, they must also be result-oriented. The manager should begin by completing the first task efficiently, on time, and with the intended consequences. This activity leads to effectiveness as well as efficiency.

Since the manager's day is mostly unstructured, wise judgment must be used in matching time with tasks. There is a difference between being busy and being productive. The effort expended should be merely a means and not an end in itself. The manager should focus on the desired results.

Individuals cannot control time; they can, however, control their behavior within timespans. Time management requires a change in habits and attitudes. There is often a discrepancy between what one does and what one should do. Time management is largely a matter of self-discipline.

The basis for an individual's value to a company is in productive time rather than total elapsed "working" time. Individuals should recognize the existence of a time management problem if they find themselves in any of the following situations: (1) wishing for more time; (2) constantly working long hours; (3) continually "fighting fires;" (4) wanting to make a larger contribution but unable to get started (Scott, 1978, p. 58).

The problem with managing time is two-dimensional since the direction of organizational influence is from top-down and at the same time, spiralling up from the lower levels of the organization. The manager not only clutters up his own job when he is ineffective but also makes it very difficult for his subordinate managers to delegate properly to their own subordinates, since he must constantly be in control and demands that they be responsive to his every whim. The inability or unwillingness to delegate is a problem for many health care administrators that multiplies by generating unnecessary but increasing anxieties. This unwillingness is a result and not a cause; it is a symptom, rather than a disease. One of the problems is that individuals are not organized themselves and therefore cannot understand the need to delegate. Delegation is not the only method of managing time, but it is an important managerial principle that must be considered in time management and, ultimately, stress reduction.

Most executives never attempt to analyze their job and break their job down into components or steps so that they can actually understand what they are being held accountable for. If they would look at what they perform over a one-week period, they would understand what is actually productive time and what other time is wasted. Most managers have little understanding of the growth potential of their position and therefore perceive their job as a neverending spiral.

## WHAT TO DO? SOME SOLUTIONS

Many positions of authority and responsibility in health care institutions are held by persons who have excellent credentials and experience in one or another medical-related specialty or discipline. Because of doing an outstanding job and being desirable employees, they are advanced and promoted to high-level positions in departments or to supervisory administrative posts. It was assumed that in moving up the ladder they somehow acquired the necessary management skills, and in some cases this may be true. For many, however, any managerial ability was learned the hard way from basic, and at times unpleasant, trial and error experiences. There is no argument with the premise that experience is indeed an excellent teacher, but having a strong educational background is a most valuable asset. Any medical professional should agree to that!

The field of health care administration is as yet young, as it is only within the past decade or so that colleges and universities have granted any sizeable number of degrees in this discipline. Today the various facets of management are an integral part of these courses of study, and thus fill an educational gap that previously existed. In this connection it is interesting to note that students in both undergraduate and graduate programs in nursing are now showing keen interest in having more exposure to management courses.

The five basic functions of management—planning, organizing, staffing, coordinating, and controlling—are very much a part of the daily routine of all health care organizations, and supervisory personnel should be knowledgeable in these important areas. The fact that health care is a highly labor-intensive industry, filling the wants and needs of dependent patients, only serves to emphasize the need for a thorough understanding and use of management skills and techniques. While the nomenclature of specific industries may vary, the basic functions of management, with slight modification, remain immutable and thus constitute what Fayol (1937, p. 101) described as one science that is equally adaptable to both private and public affairs.

Before managing others, the first step is to have the manager understand what he does in his job, in his role, and with his time. Bonoma and Slevin (1978, p. 22) have developed a model to demonstrate some ways to save time, which is shown in Figure 1-1.

Fanning and Fanning (1979, pp. 154-155) have also developed a list for managers to use in managing their time:

1. Break it up—then start only what you can finish.
2. Do the least you can.
3. Ask yourself, "Who says I have to do this?"
4. Ask yourself, "Why do I have to do this now?"
5. Wear a watch without a second hand, if you need a watch at all.
6. Learn to say "Yes!" to insistent people, but be insincere.
7. Ask yourself, "Who says I have to do this?" (Law of Shirking)
8. Tell yourself, "Ten years from now, this will seem very important." (Law of Perspective)
9. If you absolutely have to do something, set aside some time for doing it when you don't need to eat or sleep.
10. Try hard not to worry about getting things done.
11. Only buy T-shirts with pockets (otherwise you're always looking for a place to put things).
12. Don't live by slogans; thinking is better.
13. Don't think in categories; don't go by numbers.

**Figure 1-1** Time Saving Model

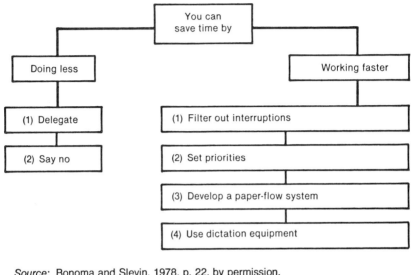

*Source:* Bonoma and Slevin, 1978, p. 22, by permission.

Edwin Bliss (1977) has enlarged upon several proven methods for managing time more effectively while achieving tasks: taking breaks, eliminating clutter, using conference calls, and saying no.

## Breaks

To work for long periods without taking a break is not an effective use of time. Energy decreases, boredom sets in, and physical stress and tension accumulate when a person stays with one thing too long. Irritability, chronic fatigue, headache, anxiety, and apathy all can be caused by failure to provide a change of pace during the working day.

A break need not be a "rest" break—indeed, switching to a different kind of work often can provide as much relief from tension as simply relaxing. Switching for a few minutes from a mental task to something physical can provide such a break. Walking around the office or around the block can serve as a quick restorative break. Changing from a sitting position to a standing position for a while can break up the monotony and provide some physical stimulus. Isometric exercises—tensing various muscles and working them against each other—can be done at your desk and are a good way to get a break from work.

Merely resting, however, is often the best course, and you should not think of a restorative break as poor use of time. Not only will being refreshed increase your efficiency, but relieving tension will benefit your health. Anything that contributes to health is good time management (Bliss, pp. 14-15).

## Clutter

Some people use clutter as a sorting device. They have a constant swirl of papers on their desks and operate on the assumption that somehow the most important matters will float to the top. This seems to work fairly well for some, and if it works, that's fine. Such people can feel straightjacketed if required to keep a tidy desk.

But in most cases, clutter works the opposite way. It hinders concentration on a single task, because your eye is constantly diverted by other things. Clutter can create tension and frustration, a feeling of being disorganized and "snowed under."

Whenever you find your desk becoming chaotic, take time out to reorganize. Make a single pile of all your papers, then go through them (making generous use of your wastebasket) and divide them into categories of priority.

Put the highest priority item from your first pile in the center of your desk, then put everything else out of sight, either on a side table or in your desk. The temptation is to leave other high-priority items on your desk so you won't overlook them. But remember, you can think of only one thing at a time, and you can work on only one task at a time, so select the most important one and focus all your attention on it (Bliss, pp. 23-24).

## Conference Calls

The most underused timesaving device, I am convinced, is the conference call.

In case you don't know (and it's surprising how many people don't), the conference call is simply a way of holding a meeting with any number of people, in almost any number of places, via telephone. You set it up simply by dialing 0 and giving the conference operator the names and phone numbers. Of course, it helps if you previously have alerted the people you intend to include, so they will be available and will have an idea of what is going to be discussed.

Many who use the conference call to bring together people in several different cities forget that it is equally valuable on a local basis.

An incidental benefit of conference calls: When people know they are going to be charged by the minute, they tend to do their homework ahead of time and are much more concise in their discussion (Bliss, pp. 34-35).

## No

Of all the timesaving techniques ever developed, perhaps the most effective is the frequent use of the word no.

You cannot protect your priorities unless you learn to decline, tactfully but firmly, every request that does not contribute to the achievement of your goals.

The tendency of many time-pressured people is to accept grudgingly new assignments in volunteer organizations, new social obligations, new chores at the office, without realistically weighing the cost in time. Such people worry about offending others—and wind up living their lives according to other people's priorities.

At work, of course, you cannot always turn down the request that you take on a job, even though you think it a waste of time. But you can win a good percentage of the time if you try. Point out to your boss how the new task will conflict with higher priority ones and suggest alternatives. If your boss realizes that your motivation is not to get out of work but to protect your time to do a better job on the really important things, you'll have a good chance of avoiding unproductive tasks. But you have to speak up (Bliss, pp. 100-101).

## MANAGERIAL SELF-ANALYSIS

Health care managers have at their disposal the following five time-use checklists that can yield insights about individual style and concern with time so that corrections can be made that will lead to a more effective and efficient operation.

*Analysis One:*

- Do I know how much time I allot to each type of task?                    _____

- Do I make sure important information is passed on and used as soon as possible?                    _____

- Do I minimize written reports?                    _____

- Do I skim reading material?                    _____

- Do I have a system to rapidly process incoming communications?                    _____

- Do I effectively use subordinates, assistants or coworkers to get better control of my time?                    _____

- Do I allocate my prime time to do important tasks?                    _____

- Do I force myself to make decisions systematically and as quickly as possible?                                           _____

- Have I worked at writing rapidly and clearly?                      _____

*Analysis Two:*

- Do I have a clearly defined set of long-range goals?               _____

- Do I have a detailed set of goals for the next three months?       _____

- Have I done something yesterday and do I plan something today to move me closer to my long-range and short-range goals?                                        _____

- Do I periodically question my objectives and reassess my priorities?                                                        _____

- Do I have a systematic method for setting my top priorities and for determining the necessary programmed steps to accomplish these top priorities?             _____

*Analysis Three:*

- Do I make a detailed schedule for each day?                        _____

- Do I make a conscious effort to compress tasks?                    _____

- Do I concentrate on high-priority items when I schedule my day, staying aware of the posteriorities I am establishing?                                                 _____

- Am I aware of what I want to accomplish next week?                 _____

- Do I have a method to remember postponed tasks?                    _____

- Do I have a way to make sure I take time to plan?                  _____

*Analysis Four:*

- Do I have a checklist for my major daily activities?               _____

- Do I review my progress at the end of each day?                    _____

- Do I set deadlines for myself and my subordinates?                 _____

- Do I make a daily measurement of my personal effectiveness?                                               _____

- Do I have a journal to record ideas, results of meetings, assignments?    _____

*Analysis Five:*

- Do I keep my desk clear?    _____
- Do I have a system to handle incoming, outgoing communications?    _____
- Am I really in control of my time? Do I determine my activities or are they dominated by crises and the priorities of other people?    _____
- Do I try to prevent unneeded information from reaching me?    _____
- Am I taking steps to prevent recurring crises?    _____
- Have I stopped any noneffective routine recently?    _____
- Do I take things with me to work on during lulls?    _____
- Do I have an effective plan to update my skills?    _____
- Do I analyze situations for time conservation possibilities?    _____

The key issues for health care managers to consider in managing their time will be addressed throughout this book. These elements include:

- planning
- delegation
- productivity
- managerial roles
- objectives and priorities
- trappings

Drucker (1954) has succinctly stated his philosophy regarding time management: Time is the scarcest resource, and unless it is managed nothing else can be managed. This perspective is essential for health care administrators seeking effectiveness and efficiency.

## REFERENCES

Adams, S., & Ponthieu, L. How administrators waste their time and what they can do about it. *Hospital Management,* August 1969, 46.

"Always late for work? You're slave of clock." *Montreal Gazette,* August 2, 1980.

Bliss, E.C. *Getting things done.* New York: Bantam Books, 1977.

Bonoma, T.V., & Slevin, D.P. *Executive survival manual.* Boston: CBI Publishing Co., 1978.

Cohen, J. (Ed.). *Readings in psychology.* London: Allen & Unwin, 1964.

Connors, E., & Hutts, J. How administrators spend their day. *Hospitals, JAHA,* Feb. 16, 1967, 46.

Drucker, P.F. *The practice of management.* New York: Harper and Row, 1954.

Drucker, P.F. *The effective executive.* New York: Harper and Row, 1967.

Fanning, T., & Fanning, R. *Get it all done and still be human.* New York: Ballantine Books, 1979.

Fayol, H. The administrative theory in the state. In L. Gulick & L. Urwick (Eds.), *Papers on the science of administration.* New York: Institute of Public Administration, 1937.

Hill, N. Where does your day go? *Supervisory Management,* May 1976, 24, 27.

Newman, P. Master time lest it master you. *Human Resource Management,* Fall 1977, 8.

Schuler, R.S. Managing stress means managing time. *Personnel Journal,* December 1979, *58*(12), 852.

Scott, R.E. Principles and techniques of time management. *Hospital Progress,* May 1978, 56, 58.

Sellar, D. Time's flying—and costs are soaring. *Montreal Gazette,* July 1980, 20.

Toffler, A. *Future shock.* New York: Bantam Books, 1972.

# Chapter 2

# Time Traps

**TIME MANAGEMENT HIGHLIGHTS**

1. Time management is a two-dimensional problem. The manager clutters up his own job when he is ineffective and makes it difficult for his subordinate managers to delegate properly to their own subordinates since he must control their actions due to his own insecurity.
2. Tension and anxiety affect the managers who waste a great deal of time in trying to reduce these conditions. They also exercise less than accurate judgment in decision making.
3. Managers attempt to halt the movement of time by employing the time trap of procrastination. The ability to overcome procrastination can be developed by minimizing past failures, accenting past successes, and setting reasonable, attainable goals.
4. Managers often get caught in an activity trap when they become so enmeshed in activity that they lose sight of why they are doing it. The activity becomes a false goal, an end in itself. The activity-centered manager is preoccupied with the volume of activities— looking busy is more important than being productive. The outcome of the activity trap in health care organizations is that purposes become subverted.
5. Ways to overcome the activity trap include:
   a. setting worthy goals
   b. getting commitment from people
   c. accepting responsibility for results
   d. supporting one's subordinates
   e. imparting a sense of mastery and satisfaction
   f. relieving employees from goal pressures

6. Management must define objectives for the organization or motivational systems will not be linked with productivity. Results are losses in profits and time.

7. The types of management time include: boss-imposed time, system-imposed time, and self-imposed time. The manager's strategy is to increase discretionary time by minimizing subordinate demands and traps.

8. We may think of time in the context of the economist's opportunity cost which can be accomplished by comparing one person's use of time with what otherwise could have been accomplished by using this same time in other ways.

9. A great deal of time is lost by the manager who does not have an agenda in dealing with time-consuming telephone calls.

10. Drop-in visitors are also time wasters who must be redirected to other sources for their communications needs.

11. Meetings and conferences often occupy a great deal of nonproductive time.

12. Managers are also held captive by "programmed tapes" which are hidden agendas that are passed on to individuals from a host of sources and dictate how time is to be spent.

13. Managers waste time by being activity oriented and not results oriented. They also impose unrealistic time estimates on activities, which creates greater stress.

14. Lack of delegation creates dissatisfaction on the part of subordinates, which results in lower organizational performance.

15. Delegation entails the setting of attainable objectives with a view of results to be determined, similar to MBO.

16. Insecurity may be a reason why a manager fails to delegate to capable subordinates. These intrapsychic factors can create conflict and stress for those involved in this complex process.

17. An effective component to delegation is the process of follow up, which may range from extremely close to laissez-faire depending upon the situation and style of manager.

18. Time management actually means less stress for individuals, which results in more efficient, satisfied and healthy employees who have an impact upon an effective organization.

Psychiatrists, psychologists, and philosophers have held varied concepts of time. Kafka (1972) described time as a series of successive instants of self-awareness organized by perception into a continuity and connected with memory. According to Eric Erikson (1956), the infant experiences time when its appetite for the mother's breast is frustrated, resulting in tension. Certain clinical phenomena give credibility to the notion that this postponement of gratification results in a trauma whose residue can be found in the psychology of later years (Schiffer, 1978, p. 11). This may help to explain adults' preoccupation with time and, often, frustrated tolerance with time.

Generally speaking, time moves slowly for the young, holding a promise of great things to come. For the imprisoned, it's a stretch to be served, just as for the bored, it's something to kill. For those maturing into adulthood, time may be a trustworthy guide, but for those who are well beyond childhood, it is an enemy to be thwarted, an unwelcome agent of transience, taking us on all too swift a journey. Indeed, for those of us over 40, it is enemy number one—a target for assassination (Schiffer, p. 13). This urgency and trauma toward time creates traps that become entrenched within our normal functioning.

It is no wonder that many individuals attempt to halt the movement of time by employing yet another trap—procrastination. Procrastination is the passionate reflection of man's heroic efforts to alter the trauma of time through an undoing of the separation from that which gave him life (Schiffer, p. 241). Freud felt there was a relationship between time and creativity. He perceived that an artist's perceptions of time and the manner in which his imagination becomes enlisted in his search for timelessness significantly determines the quality of his art (Freud, 1959). This can be projected to the health care milieu where administrators forego planning and structure for the juggling of resources which appear to be an endless alternative only to realize that their "creative" decision has them entrapped.

In discussing the relationships among motivation, leadership, and time management, Meyer (1967, p. 709) noted the following characteristics of a leader:

- is goal directed and self-motivated,
- inspires and exercises initiative,
- possesses genuine self-confidence,
- has the ability to concentrate,
- uses creativity and imagination,
- knows how to motivate others to action.

The single greatest leadership tool is the ability to overcome procrastination and thus avoid time traps. Meyer argued for the importance of self-concept, claiming that negative thinking can be reduced by

- minimizing past failures,
- mature reinterpretation of failures,

- accenting past successes,
- bolstering one's own ego by believing in oneself,
- setting reasonable, attainable goals,
- sharing responsibility,
- readiness to help.

A director of personnel for a New York corporation commented on the Freudian concept of time and creativity:

> I get my best ideas on long airplane flights, and after many years of long flights, I've just discovered why. It's because I have time to think. Artists know they need time to be creative. Why don't businesspeople, politicians and administrators recognize it? Probably it is because we don't value creativity highly enough. It doesn't have the life-or-death fullness-or-emptiness impact for us that it does for the artist. But just consider what a little bit more creativity on everyone's part could do for a corporation, a city or a hospital. Our minds have an enormous capacity for creativity, but we throw up such roadblocks. We fill our days with whatever tasks present themselves most loudly (Carlson, 1978, p. 122).

It appears that not planning for time to think is one of the greatest traps for administrators. It is not uncommon for managers to appear constantly busy while not accomplishing a thing. This may be referred to as the activity trap. This will be the first type of time trap examined in this chapter.

## THE ACTIVITY TRAP

One of the problems facing most organizations attempting to balance resources (e.g., financial, human, physical, time) is that inputs are being consumed in mass quantities, but the quality of output is less and less satisfying for the individuals who are providing the inputs to the system. Hospitals and other health services likewise make poor showings under this kind of scrutiny. The resources have been put in and the activity engaged in, but the average lifespan in this country is less than in some other countries. Why should this be happening when so much money and manpower is being poured into our health care system? (Odiorne, 1974), p. 4).

This problem has broad applicability. In business organizations, for example, the amount of money being invested in research is rising astronomically, but outputs of new products are not rising correspondingly in volume or quality. Industry studies in pharmaceuticals, in medical supplies, and in petroleum have shown that products simply are not commensurate with the resources and efforts spent to locate and develop them. There must be some explanation of this failure for organizations caught in this dilemma. The difference between successful and unsuccessful leaders and their organizations is that those who are successful are effective, efficient, and able to balance their resources, while those who are not successful, are not.

To relate this explanation to the systems approach may seem hard; however, once the explanation is couched in systems language, the problem is clear. Most people get caught in the activity trap! They become so enmeshed in an activity that they lose sight of why they are doing it, and the activity becomes a false goal, an end in itself. Successful people never lose sight of their goals and objectives, the hoped-for outputs, even while carrying on complex activities. Apparently there is a natural tendency to begin with important, clear, ideal objectives; but, in an amazingly short period of time, people become so involved in achieving their goals that they lose sight of the desired outputs and never find them clearly again. The most successful people are those who keep an eye on their objectives while they carry on complex activities. If their objectives change, they are responsive in their behavior. The less successful people continue the same behavior, even after the goals or objectives have changed (Odiorne, p. 6).

As specialization increases and knowledge workers become more abundant, there appear to be a number of individuals who have made an emotional commitment to just time, energy, and finances. Activity-centered managers are preoccupied with the volume of activities—looking busy is more important than being productive. They create a network of managers through which the activities are conducted and reinforced, as we can see in the following examples.

Some accountants function as if the entire organization were created solely for them to produce accounting reports, a substantial portion of which may be totally meaningless and useless to those for whom they are purportedly produced. Likewise, computers have created a whole host of occupations staffed with people generating information, some of which is substantially useless. Some new systems of data processing and Management Information Systems produce costly information that yields no innovations and few solutions.

One strategy for dealing with the activity problem is planning. The major contribution of people at the top should be in strategic planning, in defining long-range goals, and in answering questions such as: Where are we now? If we don't do anything differently, where will we be in five or ten years? Do we like the answer to that question? If not, what can we do about it? If the organization seems to be in extreme confusion, it may be because managers are clinging tightly to controlling operations, thereby leaving the strategic questions not only unanswered but unasked (Hutchinson, 1971). As issues become more difficult to understand, the development of new objectives may become equally complicated. At that point the chief executive officer (CEO) may get enmeshed in the activity trap, not realizing that things are not as they appear on the surface.

The lamentable outcome of the activity trap in corporations is that the purposes of the firm are subverted. The question "What are we in business for?" gets asked infrequently and accordingly is not answered often or successfully (Odiorne, 1974, p. 13). The six most efficacious factors in overcoming the activity trap, and thereby revitalizing organizations, have been described as the following (Odiorne, p. 23):

1. Setting worthy goals. For higher levels in large organizations, these are strategic goals, dealing with the basic direction and character of the organization. For operational levels and individuals, the goals are statements of conditions that will exist if the personnel are successful as members of the organization.

2. Getting commitment from people. What is required is not a personality trait but some assurance that the individual will produce specific outputs in a reasonable time frame, within defined constraints.

3. Accepting responsibility for the results of one's own behavior and, in leadership, for that of one's followers.

4. Supporting and assisting one's subordinates by providing the resources and moral support that will enable them to do their jobs.

5. Imparting a sense of mastery and satisfactory self-image to those who have behaved responsibly and produced up to their commitments.

6. Relieving employees from goal pressures. This is the final requirement of a sound, output-centered system. There must be provisions for goal-less activity for its own sake. The rest break, the vacation, the protection of leisure hours, the security of the home for private endeavors—these are essential.

Unless individuals are active, they lose a great deal of effectiveness, insight, and critical edge. Inactivity can create feelings of isolation or lead to meaningless activity. A goal is essential for finding meaning in work, even when the goal itself is not of great moment. Indeed, if a particular effort is understood to be goal-related, the suppressive effects of a lowly or even undesirable goal upon the personalities of the people engaged in working toward it are diminished. In an organization that concentrates control as close to the top as possible, rewards activity as being meritorious for its own sake, and ignores behavior that evidences subordinates' desires to set their own goals in innovative ways, there is a substantial loss of meaning in work. The reverse is also true. In organizations where the major emphasis is upon decentralized decisions, where the system encourages and rewards individuals to set goals and make commitments to them, people find significant meaning in their work. And such organizations are apt to be effective in attaining their overall objective.

The activity trap is a self-feeding mechanism. Top management loses sight of its purposes and begins to enforce on subordinates activity controls that tend to become increasingly unrelated to any useful purpose. Meanwhile, all that activity is eating up resources (money, labor, materials) and producing less and less output. "Do it my way" becomes more important than "produce our objectives" (Odiorne, p. 27).

Organizations that focus upon activity tend to decrease achievement motivation on the part of professionals. This occurs when work is viewed not so much in terms of outputs and results but in units of activity such as excessive hours of work. This situation does not foster the acceptance of responsibility on the part of the professional employee or lead to a quest for higher levels of attainment and output. Because activity itself is the target, very little meaning is attached to task achievement.

Clarence Randall, late president of Inland Steel, once observed that company presidents are lonely people. They find they must isolate themselves from their organizations, and in the process often isolate themselves from the truth. Eleven levels of management can produce a lot of filtering. It is small wonder that the top people, even in small organizations, are often deluded into acting upon "facts" that have been polished, trimmed, slanted, or even turned completely around. They are likely to make contacts not downward, but upward, with a conservative board, which leads to the establishment of policies unsuitable for changing situations. Given such deprivation of valuable information, missteps are common. When individuals are isolated from the realities of the business they actually operate, without proper data and restrained by internal and external factors from obtaining it, they often fall back on the comfortable misconception that time by itself will solve their problems. This external orientation is quite unrealistic and leads to further problems.

## THE NEED FOR GOALS

Organizations that foster activity traps do not support goal setting or related motivational efforts. As a motivational influence, goal setting is more effective than the inefficient method of prescribing activities for subordinates. The promotion of activity-centered behavior is not based upon a structured, realistic foundation, but upon imagery. Image-thinking that is simplistic in scope produces men who will adapt to the image. When these images all have the effect of reinforcing activity and of making personal goal setting productive of unfavorable consequences, activity becomes an end in itself (Odiorne, p. 68). Unless management defines objectives for the organization, motivational systems will not be linked with productivity, with the resulting loss in profits and time. When people are lucky enough to work for an organization that has goals defined in such painstaking detail that the individual can fit his own personal goals to them, the unleashed energy and ingenuity make that organization strong. The findings of behavioral scientists such as David McClelland, Frederick Herzberg, Abraham Maslow, and Rensis Likert suggest a connection between goal setting and motivation that is just beginning to be utilized by a few leaders in organization and management. In brief, these are some of their conclusions (Odiorne, pp. 70-71):

- Motivation properly starts with anticipatory goal states.

- Motivation is a possession of responsible individuals who are committed to attainment of these anticipatory future states.

- Only a very few motives are innate or natural, and they are mainly physiological (hunger, sex, and the like) rather than emotional.

- The overwhelming body of motivation is learned, secondary, social, or psychogenic, and almost all such motives are goal-directed. McClelland suggests that every motive involves two states: "a present state which redisintegrates through past learning a second stage." An objective is a potent motivator. When objectives are systematically denied, or when activity is substituted for goals, motivation declines.

- Motivation has no single cause. It changes as the more important goals are attained; it is affected by both conscious and unconscious influences, and it evolves throughout a person's life. The best insight into normal motivation comes through observation of normal persons, not of rats, cats, primates, and abnormal persons.

- Motivation improves if due attention is paid to the objective-setting process, the defining of corporate and divisional goals, the method of stating managerial and employee objectives, and the procedural problems of goal setting.

J.K. Galbraith in *The New Industrial State* (1967, pp. 135-136) proposes a general theory of motivation which prescribes four major categories of motivational explanation: (1) The individual goes toward the group goals by compulsion. (2) The acceptance of the group's goal is purchased; this Galbraith calls *pecuniary* motivation. (3) The individual may be so taken with the goals of some group that he suspends his previous personal goals and adopts those of the group as his own; in other words, he identifies. (4) The class is for the individual who sees in the group's goals a vehicle for attaining his own personal goals or a possibility of affecting the goals of the group to conform with his personal goals; this Galbraith calls *adaptive* motivation.

The activity-centered organization is void of the highest and most optimum levels of motivation and must rely on compulsion and pecuniary or other physical rewards at perhaps a constantly increasing rate to maintain what becomes meaningless work. If managers can perceive of problems to be solved as deviations from some objective, then a commitment for solution can be made by a responsible individual who is now motivated and not just activity-oriented.

The search for causes of problems is naturally backward-looking since past events must be examined. Some reasons are labeled ''causes'' and the others ''effects.'' Overemphasis on finding causation for every problem does little good; indeed, it can eventually immobilize the organization. If everyone spends time looking for causes of every untoward event, nothing new will be done. In this way the activity trap is made more viable and its strength increased. The only practical justification for finding causes is to solve a problem or to assure a better future. When the search for causes reverts to picking over past events for scandals and scapegoats, it is unworthy and unproductive work (Odiorne, 1974, p. 83). This process immobilizes the organization and adds to the already mounting wasted time and efforts.

The need to maintain activity during the problem-solving process illuminates the unrealistic need to collect an abundance of data. The strength and continuity of the activity trap is powerfully reinforced by the many pitfalls that lie before an individual or group attempting to extract significance from data. Five major sources of errors by management in interpreting data, in addition to flaws in the data itself, can be listed:

1. Managers are inundated with more information than they can possibly use.
2. High-level management tends to see only the total picture—to see things wholly and globally.
3. They mistake the essence of the issue.
4. They worship measurement, or
5. They hate measurement and worship the vague.

## THE MANAGERIAL PARADIGM

Managers can improve the quality of their supervisor-subordinate relationships. This goal helps to transmit to subordinates the optimum skills of the manager, which leads to a more effective and efficient operation and a saving of time. The following objectives are worthy of consideration:

1. The manager deals with goals and results. While the subject of methods and activities is not ignored by any means, the primary purpose of the face-to-face relationship lies in its almost spartan control over irrelevancies, a

detailed exposition and discussion of objectives, and analysis of actual results as compared with those objectives.

2. The objectives themselves are treated with care and are expanded upon until clarity and agreement are complete. The delegation of results expected is as complete as human judgment and communication skill will allow, and the assessment of results is meticulously compared with the original goals.

3. The nature of the discussions is less apt to be judgmental than affirmative, optimistic, forward-looking, and problem-centered. Discussions of "your strengths and weaknesses" are far less likely to be on the agenda than discussion of "how could we do an even better job in the future?"

4. The discussion is not what Eric Berne refers to as "parent-child" discussions, in which the boss serves in loco parentis, issuing advice and admonitions. Rather, it resembles Berne's adult-adult relationship: two grownups strike bargains and make mutual commitments. The subordinate makes promises to attempt to produce certain outcomes in the future, and the manager, in turn, is committed to certain supportive and helpful behaviors.

5. Group meetings, such as board meetings, task forces, and committees likewise concentrate upon goals, results, and mutual commitments. Unlike many staff meetings which concentrate endlessly upon activities, with the least relevant information occupying the greatest period of time, the groups focus upon target aims and very specific objectives. When ideas come to a standstill, or the path is unclear, the activity required is suggested, not as a means of suppressing or controlling members, but for clearing obstacles, providing shared knowledge, and stimulating innovation through the process of suggestion.

## FROM CHAOS TO CRISES

Larry Meares, Vice President of Human Resources for Russell, Burdsall and Ward Corporation, suggests that the application of the following principles will result in disunity, distrust, lack of commitment, and chaos (1979, pp. 473-475). This of course leads to crisis-producing dysfunctional behavior resulting in loss of productivity and time. Management usually invests a large number of unproductive workhours in correcting these problems.

1. Create distinct and visible status symbols which make everyone sensitive to the "haves" and "have nots" at various levels of the organization.

2. Refrain from installing any type of formal promotion and transfer procedure.

3. At lower levels of the organization's hierarchy, ignore seniority completely when contemplating any work-related promotion, transfer, or other reward

considerations, except where required for vacation accrual or pension vesting.
4. Communicate only mundane and elementary information.
5. Title people with levels of visible difference, e.g., the hourly or factory subordinate, as opposed to the salaried, exempt manager, and refer to them by these titles instead of by their names.
6. Deliberately refrain from the installation of position descriptions, authority parameters, or any other semblance of a performance appraisal system.
7. Encourage favoritism wherever possible.
8. Make it a public practice to discharge errant persons without employing a system of progressive consultation.
9. Provide nothing which resembles a system permitting persons to air their complaints, problems, questions, or suggestions.
10. Provide no management development or training for members of supervision and other management personnel.
11. Retain only managers who are mechanically and technically competent, but managerially deficient.
12. Establish written rules and regulations for every conceivable infraction, and impose them without flexibility on the group for whom they are intended.
13. Encourage each member of management to hire and staff all vacancies under their jurisdiction, without providing any assistance or training in how to perform such activities.
14. Maintain benefits and pay levels below the average of the competitive marketplace.
15. Follow a policy of affixing individual blame when mistakes or errors occur, and especially stress punitive measures.
16. Discourage socializing, whether on or off the job.
17. Attempt to avoid any formalized approach to planning and forecasting, since it often leads to a more stable work group, with too many participants aware of too much information.
18. Always attempt to visibly show disrespect for the dignity of the people you want to disturb or upset.
19. Make it a routine practice to promise people whatever they need or want and then conveniently forget to live up to your word.
20. It is always helpful to arrange for managers and supervisors to be caught telling untruths to each other and their employees, so take care to always plant at least one or two "whoppers" that will be naturally discovered in the course of daily events.
21. Never provide advance notice when overtime work is necessary.
22. If you have the unfortunate tendency to be outgoing and friendly, you must overcome it!

23. Always take credit for the contributions of others, and make sure they find out.
24. Do a lot of monotonous lecturing about everything.
25. Criticize everyone to everyone else.

In addition to this unique listing of things to avoid, there are many other time traps for the health care manager to consider.

## THE IMPOSITION OF TIME

It is not unusual for managers to run out of time while their subordinates are running out of assignments. This is one of the traps to look for and then avoid. Managers must increase their leverage, which will help them to multiply the value of each hour that they spend in managing "management time." Specifically, we shall deal with three different kinds of management time:

1. Boss-imposed time—to accomplish those activities that the boss requires and the manager cannot disregard without direct and swift penalty.
2. System-imposed time—to accommodate those requests to the manager for active support from peers. This assistance must also be provided lest there be penalties, though not always direct and swift.
3. Self-imposed time—to do those things which the manager originates or agrees to do himself. A certain portion of this kind of time, however, will be taken by subordinates and is called "subordinate-imposed time." The remaining time will be his own and is called "discretionary time." Self-imposed time is not subject to penalty since neither the boss nor the system can discipline the manager for not doing what they did not know he intended to do in the first place.

The manager's strategy is therefore to increase the discretionary component of his self-imposed time by minimizing or doing away with the subordinate component. He will then use the added increment to get better control over his boss-imposed and system-imposed activities. Most managers spend much more subordinate-imposed time than they even faintly realize (Oncken & Wass, 1974, pp. 75-76).

To avoid this trap, the manager must not be "imposed upon" by his subordinates, who would like nothing more than to transfer the initiative for problem solving to him. Unfortunately, both parties cannot effectively have the same initiative at the same time.

There are five degrees of initiative that the manager can exercise in relation to the boss and to the system: (1) wait until told (lowest initiative); (2) ask what to do; (3) recommend, then take resulting action; (4) act, but advise at once; and (5) act on own, then routinely report (highest initiative).

Clearly, the manager should be professional enough not to indulge himself in initiatives 1 and 2 in relation either to the boss or to the system. A manager who uses initiative 1 has no control over either the timing or content of his boss-imposed or system-imposed time. He thereby forfeits any right to complain about what he is told to do or when he is told to do it. The manager who uses initiative 2 has control over the timing but not over the content. Initiatives 3, 4, and 5 leave the manager in control of both, with the greatest control being at level 5.

The manager's job, in relation to his subordinates' initiatives, is twofold: first, to outlaw the use of initiatives 1 and 2, thus giving his subordinates no choice but to learn and master "completed staff work;" then, to see that for each problem leaving his office there is an agreed-upon level of initiative assigned to it, in addition to the agreed-upon time and place of the next manager-subordinate conference. The latter should be duly noted on the manager's appointment calendar (Oncken & Wass, p. 79).

The only way the manager can control the timing and content of his position is for him to enlarge his discretionary time by eliminating the trap of subordinate-imposed time. This objective, if successful, can be termed effective managing.

In today's organizations, with the many demands for time and attention, the available amount of discretionary time is constantly being eroded. As each extra hour or even 15 minutes becomes scarcer, it takes on added significance and value, finally resulting in what can be called "time inflation." Dealing with this notion of time inflation, that is, the constantly increasing value of one's available time relative to the demands made upon it, is not easy. There are, however, a few basic maxims concerning opportunity costs and the law of comparative advantage.

## Opportunity Costs

The initial approach is to think of time in the context of the economist's "opportunity cost," which is accomplished by comparing one person's use of time with what otherwise could have been accomplished by using this same time in other ways. This is not just setting priorities, but goes beyond that. By doing A, it is impossible to be doing B. Is the time cost for B more or less valuable than performing A? In addition, it is quite possible, given the proper data, to determine approximate, if not actual, monetary costs of alternatives. In the case of very large, complex, and expensive ventures, such as purchasing a CAT scanner or electron microscope, the use of cost-benefit analysis would, of course, be advisable.

## The Law of Comparative Advantage

The second method is a broad application of David Ricardo's 19th century law of comparative advantage. Simply stated in terms of time use, this says that each person should do that work for which he or she is relatively better qualified than someone else. It would seem to be a complete misdirection of talent for a gourmet cook to be the dishwasher in a restaurant, or for that matter, for an architect to push a wheelbarrow of bricks or cement. Yet mismatches, perhaps not as bizarre as these, do occur, and result in a total misallocation of needed resources and, relative to time use, high cost. Persons who have training and expertise in highly sophisticated specialties should be employed in jobs with responsibilities that are commensurate with their skills. To do otherwise, obviously, is a waste of time.

## UTILITARIAN TIME TRAPS

There are a great many other time traps that managers become entangled with in their quest to effectively manage their time and juggle their responsibilities. These traps include the following.

## The Telephone

The telephone, while being one of the great inventions, creates a problem since it is an interrupter that forces managers to change their style of work. Some ways of handling the telephone include:

- Have others filter your calls and handle them whenever possible.

- Encourage individuals to call other people in the organization who can handle the problem.

- Do not accept any calls when you need private time for thinking.

- Lump together all of your calls and make them at one time.

- Cut out the small talk on the telephone and get down to business.

- Have a written agenda for each multitopic phone call.

- Have all of the important information you need in front of you before making the call.

## Drop-In Visitors

Drop-in visitors are problems because they stop by to say hello and at the same time give the manager bits and pieces of grapevine information. The next time the manager looks at his watch, a half-hour or more has elapsed, with a questionable amount of essential data having been transmitted and little work done. This leads to increased frustration and a lowered feeling of job satisfaction. There are ways of handling this situation. Some suggestions are:

- Train your own manager and your subordinates to respect your time and not to drop in.
- Close your door for a period of time.
- Meet with your subordinates on a regular basis and force them to develop an agenda to be utilized.
- Avoid any instant discussion in recurring emergencies and crises. These will clear up.
- Develop an office structure and layout that permits you to communicate your attitudes toward individuals who seem to want to hang around.
- When somebody comes in to say hello, stand up and remain standing until the other person leaves.
- Suggest the next meeting be held in their office.
- Analyze why people drop in—it may be your need to talk to them that creates this problem.

## Meetings and Conferences

These create problems because we find that their productivity is low with questionable results. Meetings seem to be popular and frequent within organizations because they have been part of the communication system within the organization historically and no one has ever attempted to understand how to communicate in a one-to-one or small project group manner; therefore they exist! The following can be employed by the manager in order to make meetings more productive:

- Learn something about the group process and how to deal with small groups so that you can minimize the number of conflicts within the meeting and have more productive meetings.

- Keep the number of meetings to a small number and explore any alternatives appearing to be valid.

- Choose a time and place that will maximize attendance and have specific objectives ready.

- Have an agenda ready with specific times and responsibilities for each member to accomplish.

- Distribute the agenda prior to the meeting.

- Begin the meeting and end the meeting on time and do not allow petty interruptions.

- Make sure that each point is handled quickly and get closure on each point. It is important to accomplish the objectives of the meeting without tabling these issues for ensuing meetings.

- Abolish committees that have no basic purpose or those that have already achieved their purposes.

- Whenever possible, do not go to a meeting or call one unless it is essential for decision making and productivity. This is a good time to delegate the responsibility to an assistant to handle those aspects of the meeting that you have handled previously.

## Programmed Tapes

Programmed tapes are basically individual "prerecorded" hidden agendas that have been passed on to us by parents and other people who have had an impact on our lives. Some of these messages indicate to us how we should deal with certain issues, and we have accepted these messages without question. These tapes all possess subliminal messages regarding the management of time:

- *Tape A:* These messages discourage good time management by overstressing motion and activity. Some of the quotes that we often hear are: "Don't waste any time," "Don't just sit there, do something," "Keep busy," "Always work hard," "The longer and harder you work, the more you get done."

- *Tape B:* These tapes encourage overplanning, overcaution, or perfectionism and they include such quotes as: "Don't make any mistakes," "Anything worth doing is worth doing well," and "Always do it the right way."

- *Tape C:* These tapes discourage planning and they include statements like: "All things come to those who wait," "Good things are unexpected," "Take care of today and let tomorrow take care of itself."

- *Tape D:* These tapes are intended to discourage delegating by stating things like: "If you want a thing done right, you have to do it yourself," or "Never ask anybody to do something you wouldn't do yourself."

The problem with these tapes is that individuals have been conditioned by them for a long time and, as a result, find that they do not have the analytical insight to make any changes.

## The Problem of Procrastination

One of the more popular styles of decision-making avoidance is the art of procrastination. This avoidance is associated with the fight or flight response, a component of anxiety and stress. Managers have a fear of mistakes and their hypothesized punishments. They often avoid the making of a decision because their fantasy is that the solution to the problem will be more effective if they wait a bit before making it. They also postpone a decision by procrastinating when an effective alternative requires doing something unpleasant initially. Managers also procrastinate through indecision, which indicates a problem with prioritizing. Procrastination also occurs through the need to be perfect and to feel that everything must be performed with precision. This creates time constraints and great anxiety, since apparently the only perfect managers have been deceased for quite a while!

### BEHAVIOR TRAPS

Personal styles of behavior can also cause time loss and inefficiency within organizations.

## Late Bird

This individual seems to live by a chronically slow clock, or by no clock at all, and often claims to be the innocent victim of unexpected delays and emergencies over which there is no control. While promises are freely made, they are seldom fulfilled, and nothing is really accomplished until the last possible moment. Even then there is such a rush and flurry of excitement that mistakes are rampant. The hallmark here is procrastination, and the key words to watch for are: tomorrow, next week, or later.

## Short Cutter

A short cutter is genuinely interested in controlling the use of his time and always tries to be the first one to finish a specific task or assignment. Often speed is achieved at the expense of thoroughness and accuracy, with established routines frequently ignored or bypassed. As a result, correction of errors may take much more time than the task itself. If subsequent actions depend on the short cutter's work, the errors, if unnoticed, merely compound the difficulty and spread the problem.

## Rabbit

Generally speaking, the rabbit is closely akin to the short cutter, but different in that while usually following prescribed guidelines, tasks are performed in such a breathless manner that the end product falls short of the desired result. A lack of good allocation and scheduling of available time creates an almost frantic approach and thus precludes proper completion of the assignment, again resulting in needless errors.

## Compulsive Saver

This person acts as a miser, secretly stashing away every scrap of material or piece of information which someday may be deemed priceless. Being so preoccupied with first devising and then using an ingenious system for classifying and storing these treasures, little time is left to take care of really important matters. The result usually takes the form of a wealth of clutter, with no time for anything else.

## Firefighter

This is a common designation given to someone engaged in an occupation fraught with possibilities of sudden emergency, and the health care field certainly affords that opportunity. While most situations are of a serious nature, sometimes time and attention are focused on rather minor issues at the expense of more pressing problems, simply because it is not financially feasible to maintain an adequate staff on an emergency standby basis. While some activities may not of themselves be a matter of life or death, they nevertheless pose conditions which must be quickly resolved and thus require considerable time, effort, and imagination. Recently one administrator cited two such emergency situations: (1) finding the proper clothing for a 500-pound patient, and (2) trying to locate any living relative of an accident victim. Getting satisfactory results in these two cases was not easy, and forced an immediate reallocation of time priorities. Small emergencies must be contained and resolved promptly before they escalate into more complex situations that can only cause further disruption in the normal workload of other busy people.

## Explorer

This person, often a self-appointed committee of one, is continuously seeking answers and solutions to real or imaginary problems. Ultimately and usually quite unwittingly, he rediscovers the "wheel" which was previously tried and permanently discarded as totally unsuitable. This kind of activity not only usurps the time and energy of the explorer, but of all others who are subjected to an endless recounting of the useless activity.

## Redoer

This individual consistently makes revisions and corrections. Valuable time is lost because of an apparent lack of knowledge or understanding of what is expected. This may be due in part to poor interpersonal communication, or an inability or even unwillingness to try to comprehend instructions or explanations. Redoing work wastes this worker's time as well as that of all of those who are kept waiting for the final change or correction. Promotion of a zero defects program should help the redoer realize the need and importance of doing things right the first time.

While these descriptions may seem to be severe and harshly drawn caricatures, they do serve the intended purpose of pointing out some attitudes and working habits that commonly exist and that flagrantly abuse the use of time. Many more stereotypes could be added, but it will be left to the reader to recognize them in their various forms and hopefully to initiate the required action to eliminate, or at least minimize, such practices, particularly the effect on the time of other workers.

## PAPERWORK AND RED TAPE

Managers who don't know how to cope properly with paperwork tend to fall into the following four categories (Dreilinger, 1980, p. 22):

*Doers:* They tend to do too much of their own paperwork. Results: Work group morale suffers. Subordinates never get any juicy assignments. Moreover, doers can't be promoted because they're the only ones who know how to do the important work.

*Delegators:* They are the opposite of doers. They delegate too much without training or monitoring their staff sufficiently. Results: Work isn't done properly; it's frequently late.

*Delayers:* They typically wait until the last minute. They claim to work best under pressure, but there's never enough time to recheck work or consider more effective alternate courses of action. Results: Work is often late and of slapdash quality.

*Dumpers:* They neglect paperwork because they believe it isn't important. They tend to toss memos and reports without reading them. Results: Dumpers frequently make bad decisions based on intuition rather than facts. They also often don't know what's going on outside their immediate spheres of activity.


## THE CURRENT STATE OF THE ART: A WRAP-UP

1. Managers often complain that they do not have enough time to breathe, yet everyone has all the time needed—which is the great paradox of time.
2. Managers rarely understand just how they spend their time since their perceptions may become distorted when time is compressed and when they are experiencing stressful situations. This dilemma can be examined through a personal time analysis based on a daily log of activities for a period of at least one week. This will help the manager understand how he is allocating his time resources.
3. An effective time management device is for managers to avoid surprise and anticipatory action. This forces the use of planning, in an attempt to determine result priorities before any action is unnecessarily undertaken. Effective planning also results in purposeful objectives that create priorities and indicate to the manager a sequential order of tasks. Concentration can be focused on achieving essential objectives within a prioritized deadline, which helps to overcome indecision, vacillation, and procrastination.
4. In most areas of organized human endeavor, a critical few efforts (around 20 percent) usually produce the bulk of the results (around 80 percent). This principle is referred to as the "Pareto Principle" or the "20/80 Law."
5. Managers also seek to achieve the optimum balance of efficiency and effectiveness. They may feel that effort will tend to be ineffective if performed on the wrong tasks at the wrong time or without intended consequences.
6. Managers waste a great deal of time by becoming activity oriented and not results oriented, which impedes effectiveness.
7. Managers may impose unrealistic time estimates on their activities, which create stress for them. They tend to forget that everything takes longer than anticipated.
8. Managers usually live with a constant struggle between what they consider to be urgent and what they consider to be important.

9. Managers are conditioned to overreact to apparent problems and become too involved in firefighting and crisis management, which causes anxiety, affects their judgment, and results in improper decisions resulting in further stress for them.

10. When managers fail to perform a problem analysis and distinguish symptoms from causes, a great deal of effort is wasted as well as time, which leads to further overreaction in the attempt to compensate.

11. Managers do not often envision any alternative solutions to a problem. This feeling of helplessness creates indecision and ultimately procrastination. This cycle creates more tension while creating greater stress.

12. When managers do not delegate total responsibility and authority to subordinates to complete a whole task, this creates dissatisfaction on the part of their subordinates who ultimately sabotage the manager's efforts.

13. Managers must be able to organize and utilize time effectively in assignments. Managers who cannot clarify their own responsibilities affect their subordinates by creating ambiguous, confused situations.

14. Some managers are unable to say no to others who demand their time and expertise. This may be due to lack of awareness, to a need to help others, or to a fear of offending other people. Some even believe that saying yes to everyone enhances their prospects for promotion and upward mobility in the organization. Some of these managers are so insecure and possess such low self-esteem that they feel they must always say yes to immediate demands. Their fallacious reasoning is that those individuals in the organization who are making instant demands of them will think much more highly of them for dropping everything and responding and, therefore, they will ultimately be viewed in a much more positive way. This management philosophy and style leads to failure for all who are involved.

**REFERENCES**

Carlson, D.G. Time to think. *Personnel Journal,* March 1978, *57*(3).

Dreilinger, C. Paperwork style and managerial effectiveness. *Management Review,* January 1980.

Erikson, E. The problem of ego identity. *Journal of the American Psychoanalytical Association,* 1956, *4,* 56-121.

Freud, S. *Creative writers and day dreaming.* Standard Ed. (Vol. 9). London: Hogarth Press, 1959.

Galbraith, J.K. *The new industrial state.* Boston: Houghton-Mifflin, 1967.

Hutchinson, J.G. *Management strategy and tactics.* New York: Holt, Rinehart and Winston, 1971.

Kafka, J.F. Panel report on the experience of time. *Journal of the American Psychoanalytical Association,* 1972, *20,* 650-667.

Meares, L.B. A long-range model for organizational chaos at any level. *Personnel Journal,* July 1979, *58*(7), 473-475.

Meyer, P.J. Motivation's triple impact on business management. *The Commercial and Financial Chronicle,* August 24, 1967, *206.*

Odiorne, G.S. *Management and the activity trap.* New York: Harper and Row, 1974.

Oncken, W., Jr., & Wass, D.L. Management time: Who's got the monkey? *Harvard Business Review,* November/December 1974, *52*(6).

Schiffer, I. *The trauma of time: A psychoanalytical investigation.* New York: International Universities Press, 1978.

# Chapter 3

# Effective Time Utilization

## TIME MANAGEMENT HIGHLIGHTS

1. The primary step in developing a program of time management is to find out how available time is being used. This can be done by the keeping of a log or diary based upon a convenient and pertinent time interval.
2. The health care manager can borrow an analytical technique from inventory control to determine the proportionate time use of each work characteristic as a percentage of total available time.
3. It is essential to understand delegation as an achievement by a manager of definite, specified results which have been previously determined on the basis of a priority of needs, by empowering and motivating subordinates to accomplish all or part of the specific results for which the manager has full accountability.
4. When delegating tasks to subordinates, a key item to consider is the development of a time system for subordinates, and the objectives to be achieved which are to be determined by joint negotiation between the manager and the subordinate.
5. A decline in productivity may be traced to lower satisfaction due to failure on the part of the health care manager to delegate. Confusion and lost efficiency can be minimized by delegating a specific assignment to only one capable subordinate rather than requiring responses from several. The manager has the option to delegate all or delegate some or delegate none.
6. Proper delegation develops the essential skills of subordinates, enriches the job, creates better morale, reduces turnover, and encourages initiative.
7. Organizational health care settings moderate the effects of delegation on the outcome and have direct effects upon outcome. In

traditional settings, delegation decreases performance while effecting performance. However, in the modern organization, delegation increases performance.

8. Flexible work hours is a system to consider in which personnel are permitted to choose the hours they wish to work as long as they work a specified number of hours each budget period. In flextime, work performance seems to be more efficient due to the reduction in numbers of days lost and reduction in cost for a given output. Some advantages include organizational improvements, reduction in travel time allocation for employees due to peak rush hours, and so forth.

9. The failure to delegate indicates that the real issue may not be intellectual or cognitive, but may be a psychological problem which manifests itself emotionally in dysfunctional behavior.

10. The higher a manager is located in the hierarchy, the more he tends to be oriented to the future with regard to time and planning. This is another reason for actualizing delegation so that this manager will be able to fulfill planning, management, and assessment activities with regard to their potential for future action.

11. Problems appear when managers become overwhelmed by inaccurate perceptions. As a result of this, they spend a great deal of time experiencing anxiety and stress, which cuts into their productivity by demanding much of their energy in fighting the wrong battle.

12. Managers who solve problems intuitively feel this is the only safe way to achieve effectiveness and success. To delegate would be a greater personal problem for them since it would hamper this initial success pattern which is historically anchored.

13. Lack of trust is largely to blame for nondelegation initially and may be a major source of overmanagement and mismanagement by health care administrators who believe they are actually delegating by tightly controlling their subordinates and not giving them any decision-making responsibilities and freedom. The second time a manager delegates to the same subordinates will usually require half the time that the initial delegation process took.

14. One of the best ways to manage the effectiveness of time allocation is by the process of follow up as a control device. The amount of control that a manager exercises in the follow up to a delegated task is often determined by the unique personality of the manager, his style, the personality and style of his subordinates, and the nature of the task itself.

Whenever a senior executive—whether in business, health care, government, or the academic world—tells me that he controls more than half of his work hours, I am reasonably certain that he actually has no idea where his time goes. For "discretionary time" is one of the scarcest and most precious of commodities. It is the time which an executive has at his own judgment on matters that are truly important. In working with dozens of businessmen, I have seldom found a senior officer who controls as much as 25 percent of his time. And the higher up in the organization an executive is, the larger the share of his time which is *not* under his control, and is not spent productively (Drucker, 1966, p. 56).

This statement by Drucker portrays the plight of the manager with regard to managing the unique resource, time. Time is fascinating, since its supply is completely inelastic. Drucker has also commented that the best way to increase individuals' effectiveness is to improve their utilization of time.

Managers are usually concerned about time utilization from the perspective of "how to do it." Time management in this context is viewed as a series of principles to be faithfully followed. Such principles are important rules of thumb and can be used where applicable. However, an additional dimension is required for managers to be completely effective in the utilization of time. This dimension is the comprehension of the *value* of time. Without a conscious realization of the value of managerial time, effective time utilization will not necessarily follow from adherence to principles of time efficiency (Jackson & Hayen, 1974, p. 753). Most executives don't know this. One health care manager, for example, was absolutely certain that he divided his working hours into three equal parts—one third spent with his medical staff, one third with administrators, and the rest devoted to community activities. But when an assistant decided to take a detailed record of what the manager actually did during a month of activities, he discovered that he spent almost no time on any of these areas! In fact, the record showed that he spent most of his time as an auxiliary dispatcher, keeping track of only those activities he knew personally and bothering the staff with phone calls about them. His intervention merely wasted the other administrators' time as well as his own. When he first saw the time log he refused to accept the facts as presented.

## WHERE DID THE TIME GO?

For centuries human beings have been intrigued by the idea of keeping track of time and have devised a number of ingenious systems and intricate devices intended to measure it.

In some situations, very exact time measurement is of the utmost importance. This is particularly true in astronomy, where a special brand of "sidereal" time has been developed and adopted. Another instance occurs in navigation, where a chronometer is necessary to accurately indicate Greenwich Mean Time. Still another need for exact time measurement occurs in competitive sports, where tenths of a second are precisely monitored by electronic stopwatches. In the health care field, similar careful measurement of elapsed time is required for the administration of medications or exposure of patients to highly sophisticated diagnostic and therapeutic techniques.

The complicated and demanding schedules that encompass both work and personal situations necessitate the proper use of time for efficiency and simplicity. Individuals who conform to an imposed established time pattern often start each workday by responding to the insistent and impatient persuasion of an alarm clock or radio. Then, having arrived at our place of employment, we all may be greeted by a robotlike timing device which quite impartially notes, by stamping a card, each arrival and later departure.

Whether we like it or not, mechanisms such as these establish limits of sleep and productivity, work and leisure, and in fact become the arbitrators of individual and collective time use.

Waiting for a special day, such as a holiday or the start of a vacation, can seem to take an eternity, yet once it occurs the time usually passes so quickly that it is often over when it seems to have only just begun. The time reference quickly shifts from comments like "I'm counting the days" to "The time just flew. Why did it have to end so soon?" What has happened, of course, is that one's perception of the passage of time has changed as a result of replacing a desired expectation with an actual realization.

For individuals in work environments, time may appear to have widely varying dimensions. For those who have jobs that they consider unpleasant, minutes may drag on at an almost imperceptibly slow pace, provoking comments such as "I wish I could go home!" while for others who are enjoying a work experience, hours slip by all too fast. Here one might say, "Is it two o'clock already? I forgot to have lunch!"

A wide range of variables may influence a person's use of time. Among others, these include:

- the individual
- the job
- other workers
- the organization
- the work environment

But, because this book is solely concerned with the management of time, a consideration of the impact of these and other factors is left to others involved in personnel administration, interpersonal relationships, and organizational development.

## THE LOG

The first step in developing a program of time management is simply to find out how available time is really being used. All that is necessary is to get the answer to "What did I do today?" This need not be a complicated or long drawn-out procedure, but should be done regularly and promptly to ensure as much accuracy as possible. Otherwise, the results may generate inadequate and unreliable information, which becomes the basis for analysis and future guidelines and direction. Two decades ago, Peter Drucker recognized the need for executives to effectively use their time and made this comment: "But one cannot even think of managing one's time unless one first knows where it goes" (Drucker, 1967, p. 35).

Probably the easiest way to find out how time is used is by keeping a simple log or diary based on some convenient and pertinent time interval. The best way to do this is by recording work incidents in the log. This helps to identify patterns of interaction and ways we use time. These incidents are not *crises* but simply any change in what we are doing at our jobs. From this method we can find out whether the incidents are being interrupted, why, and for how long. While half-hour timespans are recommended, either shorter or longer periods may be more appropriate. Initially, the number of work weeks logged should allow for the inclusion of as wide a scope of recurring and nonrecurring activities as possible. For some people, two weeks may be enough, although this is merely an arbitrary limit and should be adjusted as necessary to fit specific needs. This is essential for health care administrators who are encouraged to delegate, so that they can invest their time in other more viable managerial activities.

## Work Characteristics

Because it is often difficult and at times confusing to identify and isolate the performance of some activities and functions (particularly planning, organizing, staffing, coordinating, and controlling), it is most helpful to fall back on using basic work characteristics that can be clearly defined and classified. Seeking answers to When? Where? With Whom? and How? should, in general, produce sufficient hard data for later evaluation.

Exhibits 3-1 and 3-2 contain listings of many options that may be selected and incorporated into the design of a daily log reporting form for either one specified job or for use by a group of people having similar duties and responsibilities. In each situation the mix of work characteristics should be appropriate to the job, not merely to seeking information of little or no value. Each log may possibly be unique, as it is important to decide beforehand what kind of specific information is desired. Exhibit 3-2 is an example of a daily time log generally suitable for a wide variety of jobs. Although the listing of suggested work characteristics and the sample time log are intended to be self-explanatory, the following comments may be helpful.

*When?* "When" establishes the exact time a work characteristic occurs or is performed, its duration, and its frequency of occurrence. As noted in Exhibit 3-1, timespans may be set in an arbitrary manner, although half-hour periods are recommended.

*Where?* Within the "where" category, it must be decided what locations or places are important in terms of time use. For some a simple "in" or "out" might be sufficient, while for others, something like "at a scheduled meeting" would be of greater interest.

*With Whom?* In the "with whom" grouping, time spent with persons listed as subdivisions of wider classifications may be further refined and expanded to reveal specific information; for example, medical personnel may be broken into surgeons, attending physicians, R.N.s, L.P.N.s, and so forth. In like manner, community members can be separated into clergy, the media, local community representatives, and so forth.

*How?* The "how," or performance, segment indicates what is actually being done, and it might be advantageous to further identify reading within "paperwork" and designate telephoning as one element of "conversing."

Some overlap can be expected, and this can be minimized by encouraging the recorder to enter clarifying comments in an extra space designated "open end." Entries are made by placing checkmarks in the appropriate boxes, with the dominant time use indicated in each time slot. Occasionally this may pose a problem due to a high incidence of interruptions or the inability of the person who is logging time to differentiate any single work characteristic. In such situations, a mark entered in the "fragmented" column indicates that no principal work characteristic occurred during the time period.

It should be emphasized that this type of log permits considerable latitude in design, depending on the wants and needs of the individual or the organization. For example, columns for personal time, scheduled breaks, or meals may easily be included, as required. Once the time log is underway and some insights have been gained, a Management Activities Summary Sheet like the one shown in Exhibit 3-2 can be completed to reflect the typical day for managerial activities. This sheet can then be used to identify the most and least effective incidents that require behavior change and even delegation!

**Exhibit 3-1** Work Characteristic Options for a Time Log

I. *When?* (Time Interval)

   1. How
   2. 30 minutes
   3. 15 minutes
   4. Other

II. *Where?* (Location)

   1. In employing institution
      a. own office
      b. other office
      c. scheduled meeting
      d. other

   2. Outside employing institution
      a. travelling
      b. at home
      c. scheduled meeting, convention
      d. other

   3. Other

III. *With Whom?* (Specific person or persons)

   1. Alone

   2. Administrative Personnel
      a. superior
      b. colleague, peer
      c. subordinate
      d. other

   3. Medical Personnel
      a. physician
      b. registered nurse
      c. resident
      d. other

**Exhibit 3-1** continued

4. Department Head (by activities?)

5. Patient

6. Community member
   a. clergy
   b. press
   c. government official
   d. patient family
   e. other

7. Volunteer and Auxiliary Group

8. Vendor representative

9. Regulatory agency representative

10. Association representative

11. Third party representative

12. Consultant—legal, accounting

13. Patient advocate—ombudsman

14. Board member

15. Other


IV. *How?* (Performance of Work)

1. Conversing
   a. physically, face to face
   b. telephoning
   c. participation in scheduled meeting
   d. other

2. Paperwork
   a. reading
   b. writing
   c. numerical calculations
   d. other

**Exhibit 3-1** continued

3. Observing
   a. individual (by activity?)
   b. group effort (by activity?)
   c. other

4. Thinking
   a. evaluating
   b. deciding
   c. other

5. Inspecting

6. Other

**Exhibit 3-2** Management Activities Summary Sheet

1. Number of incidents:                    _____

2. Average duration (minutes):             _____

3. Number of interruptions:                _____

4. Location of incidents                   _____
   My office                               _____
   Superior's office                       _____
   Subordinate's office                    _____
   Other                                   _____
   Total                                   100%

5. Allocation of time:

**Exhibit 3-2** continued

| Who | How | What | Function |
|---|---|---|---|
| Superiors ____ | Formal Meeting ____ | Acctg/Fin. ____ | Planning ____ |
| Peers ____ | Informal Meeting ____ | Mktg/Sales ____ | Organizing ____ |
| Subordi-nates ____ | Telephone ____ | Production ____ | Staffing ____ |
| Other Internal ____ | Social ____ | R&D ____ | Directing ____ |
| External Contact ____ | Reading ____ | Public Rela-tions ____ | Coordinating ____ |
| Alone ____ | Writing ____ | General Manage-ment ____ | Reporting ____ |
| Other ____ | Reflecting ____ | Other ____ | Budgeting ____ |
| | Other ____ | | Other ____ |

6. Now answer these important questions:   YES   NO
   a. Do you have too many incidents a day to man-age your job effectively?
   b. Are your incidents too short to be effective?
   c. Do you have too many interruptions?
   d. Are you spending your time in the wrong loca-tions?
   e. Would you like to change your time allocations
      —who?
      —how?
      —what?
      —function?
   f. Can you do more delegation?

Every "yes" answer requires action and also represents an opportu-nity for time saving.

*Source:* Adapted from Bonoma and Slevin, 1978, p. 18, by permission.

## Conducting the Survey

Once the logs have been prepared, and preferably pretested to correct problems, the next step is to start recording actual time use. Ideally, the entries should be made immediately following each time interval, but in any event, not later than the end of the work day. After completing the desired number of daily logs, the total amount of time devoted to each work characteristic is determined by totalling all the individual checkmark entries, by columns. Average time, or average percentage of total elapsed time, may be computed by simple arithmetic. Each person who completes a time log should try to be as accurate and objective as possible. In some situations, a coworker or subordinate may be in a better position to record time use than the person actually performing the work!

## Analysis

By borrowing a technique from inventory control, it is possible to determine the proportionate time use of each work characteristic in health care management as a percentage of the total available time. This procedure, commonly found in purchasing management, is used for inventory control and is based on the idea that a small percentage of products account for the largest percentage of dollar volume or value of inventory. These are known as A items. Conversely, a large percentage of items, comprising the smallest percentage of volume or value, are known as C items. Those in between the extremes are, as expected, B products.

The ABC analysis can be applied to time management, and is a method of showing an individual's time profile. While it is also adaptable to "where" and "with whom" categories, Figure 3-1 analyzes eight "how" work characteristics by listing hypothetical percentages of average weekly time use. For example, 12 of a total of 40 hours were spent in meetings; therefore 30 percent of total average hours was used for this activity. After percentages for each characteristic have been calculated, they are ranked in descending order from largest to smallest, thus forming a profile of actual time use. Those characteristics whose percentages total 25 percent of the total time are considered in the A grouping. In this case, meeting and telephoning ranked 1 and 2 and constituted 2/8 or 25 percent of the eight characteristics measured. These two accounted for a cumulative average of 55 percent of the available time.

The C activities would, of course, be just the opposite. Reading, travelling, thinking, inspecting, and other amount to 5/8 or 62½ percent of the characteristics measured and, in this illustration, use 25 percent of total average time. Writing is a B item, as it demands only a relatively moderate percentage of time.

In inventory control, A items are deserving of the most attention, while C items should have the least. Applying this convention, the ABC Analysis Chart clearly indicates how an individual apportioned time and assigned priorities. Do presently

**Figure 3-1** ABC Time Analysis

From time log entries compute average time used by job characteristics and/or functions, and rank in descending order.

Example: based on 40 hours.

| Characteristic | | Average number of hours | Percent of time | Cumulative percent of time | |
|---|---|---|---|---|---|
| 1. Meeting ⎤ 2/8=25% | | 12 | 30 | 30 ⎤ A 55% | |
| 2. Telephoning ⎦ | | 10 | 25 | 55 ⎦ | |
| 3. Writing | 1/8=12½% | 8 | 20 | 75 ⎤ B 20% | |
| 4. Reading ⎤ | | 4 | 10 | 85 ⎤ C 25% | |
| 5. Travelling ⎥ | | 3 | 7½ | 92½ | |
| 6. Thinking ⎥ 5/8=62½% | | 1 | 2½ | 95 | |
| 7. Inspecting ⎥ | | 1 | 2½ | 97½ | |
| 8. Other ⎦ | | 1 | 2½ | 100 ⎦ | |

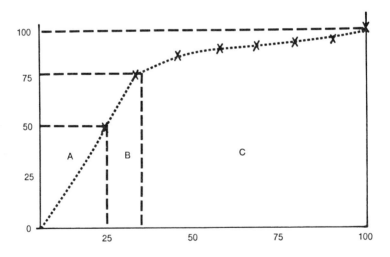

A = 25% of characteristics use 55% of time ⎤
B = 12½% of characteristics use 20% of time ⎦ A + B use 75% of time
C = 62½% of characteristics use 25% of time

designated A work characteristics really belong in C? Do some C activities deserve A status? Is time being used to its best advantage?

Benefits that result from an ABC Analysis lie primarily in the graphic portrayal of the proportion of time devoted to various work characteristics. The results may be unexpected and enlightening by revealing information that might otherwise not be so apparent. The chart thus mirrors what really happened, and provides a basis for possible evaluation and adjustment.

Use of time logs and subsequent analysis as suggested cannot by itself correct misdirected use of time or eliminate chance events that negate the most carefully thought out plans. The keeping and analyzing of a time log will, however, bring into sharp focus how time is actually spent. It provides a way to confirm one's own suspicions of excessive time use. Was a two-hour meeting with subordinates necessary? Could some items on the agenda have been handled in another way? If there had been no meeting or a shorter meeting, could the time have been used to better advantage? Do these people have two hours for such a meeting? An example can help to clarify this:

Some years ago a health care administrator was a member of an organization which held a three-hour monthly staff meeting at which attendance was compulsory. True to form, the meeting lasted about three hours, seldom ending much before or after the announced four o'clock. Quite suddenly, because of an urgent need to complete a special project, the workload of the chairman of the hospital board increased substantially. The traditional monthly meetings were abandoned in favor of one meeting each quarter, supplemented by interim written reports. Eventually the written reports appeared less frequently and were reduced in size from 30 to less than 10 pages! As a result of the new crises, time constraints were more effectively managed by prioritizing responsibilities.

Once time analysis is done on a continuing basis, principles of work simplification can be applied to make time expenditure more effective. It may be difficult to admit that one has been wasting time or not using it to the maximum advantage, but acceptance of this fact is necessary before any change can be made. Therefore, the self analysis checklist given in Exhibit 3-3 should be answered honestly. After answering these questions, the manager should compare his answers with the suggested "best" answers given in Table 3-1, assigning the indicated scores to each response. If the total score is above 25, available time is being used well. For a score below 15, time is being ineffectively managed and corrective actions should be taken immediately.

**Exhibit 3-3** Time Management Self Analysis

|  | Almost Never | Some-times | Often | Almost Always |
|---|---|---|---|---|
| 1. I keep a written log of how I spend the major portions of my working day. | | | | |
| 2. I schedule my least interesting tasks at a peak time when my energy is at its peak. | | | | |
| 3. I review my job and delegate activities that someone else could do just as well. | | | | |
| 4. I have time to do what I want to do and what I should do in performing my job. | | | | |
| 5. I analyze my job to determine how I can combine or eliminate activities. | | | | |
| 6. Actions that lead to short-run objectives take preference over those that might be more important over the long pull. | | | | |
| 7. My boss assigns more work than he thinks I can handle. | | | | |
| 8. I attack short-time tasks (answering phone calls, reading correspondence, etc.) before projects taking a long time. | | | | |
| 9. I review the sequence of my job activities and make necessary improvements. | | | | |
| 10. I arrange task priorities based on the importance of task goals. | | | | |

Personal Score _____

*Source:* J.H. Jackson and R.L. Hayen, "Rationing the Scarcest Resource: A Manager's Time." Reprinted with permission, *Personnel Journal,* October 1974, p. 754.

**Table 3-1** Suggested Best Use of Managerial Time

| Item | Almost Never | Sometimes | Often | Almost Always |
|------|------|------|------|------|
| 1. | 2 | 3 | 2 | 1 |
| 2. | 0 | 1 | 2 | 3 |
| 3. | 0 | 1 | 2 | 3 |
| 4. | 0 | 1 | 2 | 3 |
| 5. | 2 | 3 | 2 | 1 |
| 6. | 2 | 3 | 2 | 1 |
| 7. | 3 | 2 | 1 | 0 |
| 8. | 3 | 2 | 1 | 0 |
| 9. | 1 | 2 | 3 | 2 |
| 10. | 0 | 1 | 2 | 2 |

*Source:* J.H. Jackson and R.L. Hayen, "Rationing the Scarcest Resource: A Manager's Time." Reprinted with permission, *Personnel Journal,* October 1974, p. 754.

## Explanation of "Best" Time Utilization

*Item 1.* The suggested best answer to keeping a written log on activities is "sometimes." The successful manager will recognize that this activity has merit when it comes to eliminating redundant or useless effort, but he should realize that he may not need to record every day. A time consciousness developed through formal analysis will encourage an informal continuing review.

It is entirely possible to become preoccupied with accounting for how each minute is spent and lose sight of the original purpose of time analysis—to become a more efficient manager. One could be in the position of spending more time looking for wasted time than can be justified.

*Item 2.* The suggested best answer to scheduling least interesting tasks when energy is highest is "almost always." Managers spend most of their time on activities which interest them, followed by those which they do well, which are pleasurable, and which are forced upon them, and tend to put off until last those activities which are least interesting. The more pleasurable tasks should be handled at the end of the day when energy is depleted. The effective manager will attack those uninteresting (and probably more difficult) tasks when his personal energies are at their peak.

*Item 3.* The suggested best answer for delegating activities is "almost always." The logic in this reasoning is found in the words "someone else could do it just as well." The effective manager is not normally concerned with doing a job perfectly. Rather, he is interested in an optimal quality level which is arrived at by trading off quality with cost. He is interested in doing the job "well enough."

Many "professionals-turned-manager" are victimized in this regard by their own inquisitive minds. They tend to feel they must do the highest quality work possible; that tolerances must be extremely close, even though this is not required and is very expensive to attain.

*Item 4.* "Almost always" is the suggested best answer to having sufficient time to do what is needed. If the manager is complying with the principles in Items 2 and 3, the time should be available as needed.

*Item 5.* The suggested best answer is "sometimes" to managerial job analysis and combining of activities. As in the answer to Item 1, a real time consciousness will dictate that this activity be performed occasionally, but it is not necessary for formal analysis on a constant basis.

*Item 6.* The suggested best answer regarding the relative preference of short-run objectives over long-run goals is "sometimes." It must be recognized that although many people feel the long haul is the important objective, and more immediate objectives should be subjected to the long-run, this is not always true. The most desirable situation is the attainment of short-run objectives concomitant with long-run objectives. It is important to realize that while long-run goals must be served (sometimes at the expense of short-run objectives), if the short-run is *not* attended to, the long-run will never transpire.

*Item 7.* The suggested best answer to the assigning of an excessive work load by the boss is "almost never." The assumption of such behavior on the part of a superior is to assume personality quirks of some sort. However, given a normal supervisor and a greater frequency response to this question, it may be an indication that the manager's boss believes he is wasting time doing unnecessary tasks.

*Item 8.* "Almost never" is also the suggested best answer to attacking short-time duration tasks before long-time duration projects. The ten most common time problems are essentially of a short-time nature. It is entirely possible for the manager to spend his entire day handling little details, while trying to lay out blocks of time to do the big jobs. The catch is that the little jobs are recurring. The phone will always ring; the mail will always come in. These things simply do not go away unless they are made to go away, and blocks of time are essential for completing large projects. The theory behind the successful handling of this problem is that the little jobs tend to evaporate if not tended to.

*Item 9.* In reviewing the sequence of job activities, the proposed best answer is "often." The proper sequencing of job activities is all-important to the success of long-range goals. Without frequent reviews of this nature, the timing of long-range projects may be affected. The common use of the PERT/CPM method in industry today reflects this need. PERT/CPM is nothing more than a method for requiring the manager to properly sequence his activities. This kind of critical path analysis is useful in many instances and can be used quickly and easily with little practice.

*Item 10.* The suggested best answer to arranging task priorities based on task goals is "almost always." If you don't know where you are going, almost any path will take you there. A manager might be inclined to pursue those tasks which are of less than top priority unless he remains aware of the goals of those less important tasks (Jackson & Hayen, 1974, p. 755).

The purpose of this analysis was to enlighten managers about the most commonly made time management mistakes. A consciousness of time and respect for it leads to its more efficient and effective use as a resource. Once the manager has acquired the "habit" of performing self-analysis, he is ready for the systematic management of the actual working hours. The following diagnostic questions can be asked by the manager of him/herself for further insight into time management:

1. What am I doing that really does not need to be done at all—by me or by anyone else?
2. Which of the activities on my time log can be handled by someone else just as well, if not better?
3. What do I do that wastes the time of others?

These three diagnostic questions should be considered by every manager. Managers must be concerned with time wasting that results from poor management and deficient organization. Their first task is to identify the time wasters that follow from lack of system or foresight. The symptom to look for is the recurrent "crisis." Such a crisis can be prevented or reduced to a routine that assistants can handle. An example of mismanagement of time in the area of data malfunction portrays this:

The director of a large hospital was plagued for years by phone calls from doctors asking him to find beds for patients who had to be hospitalized. The admissions people "knew" there were no empty beds. Yet the administrator almost invariably found a few. The floor nurse was aware of them and so were the people in the front office who presented departing patients with their bills. The admissions people, however, were relying on a "bed count" made every morning at five o'clock—while the great majority of the patients were sent home in midmorning after the doctors had made rounds. All that was needed to put this right was to channel to the admissions office an extra carbon copy of each chit floor nurses sent the front office on patient departure.

## THE NEED TO DELEGATE

Delegation is an essential method and philosophy by which the health care manager can gain time. Delegation is the achievement by a manager of definite, specified results—previously targeted by an analysis of need priorities—by empowering and motivating subordinates to accomplish all or part of those results. The specific results for which the subordinates are accountable are clearly delineated in advance in terms of output required and time allowed, and the subordinates' progress is monitored continuously during that time period (McConkey, 1974).

This description highlights the setting of objectives with a view to the results to be determined, the priorities that are necessary, and the analysis of objectives into action plans and steps that can be delegated to subordinates. This also necessitates a review system to determine how progress is going in reaching these objectives. Delegation as described is certainly different from the assigning of tasks, but many managers have a difficult time in understanding this concept. When the manager assigns a task, the subordinate assumes the responsibility but has no authority and little accountability. This has been one of the classical management dilemmas. When a manager delegates, the subordinate assumes responsibility *and* authority and therefore is fully accountable. While managers are concerned about the risk involved in delegating, there is very little risk in passing down decision making until final action is to be taken and that can certainly be handled by the manager personally.

Managers who are perplexed about the delegation process are encouraged to examine their greater concerns about the management of time. It is easy to identify which managers have a difficult time delegating because some of them are overcontrolling; they take much of the work home at night, they are under constant pressure and criticism from their subordinates, they lack clear policies, they are slow in decision making, they possess a limited span of control, and they usually quote what their own supervisor desires to justify their actions. As a result of these factors, their efforts appear to be quite disorganized. When delegating tasks to subordinates, a key item to consider is the development of a time system for subordinates, as well as identification of the objectives to be achieved, both of which are to be determined by joint negotiation between the manager and the subordinate. When objectives are to be achieved via delegation, it is necessary to determine what priority the objectives have. The objectives and activities must be so specified that the subordinate understands what is essential and what should be accomplished by him in attempting to achieve the goals of his organization, fulfill the needs of his supervisor, and at the same time fulfill his own needs. This is the proper satisfaction mix usually recommended in organization behavior theory and practice.

In looking at delegation, it is important to note that the essence of an effective management system is not that the manager do the job himself, but that he delegate the job and its meaningful components to a capable subordinate. Managers cannot solve all time pressure problems by funnelling everything into the arena of a subordinate, abdicating their own responsibilities, and then assuming that the matter is closed. But at the same time, the manager cannot hope to keep tight, close control over every activity that goes on within his domain. It appears that some middle of the road approach is needed in order to combine the ease and confidence that accrues with having a positive feeling for your subordinates and basic operation. The delegation of an operation and assignment to an individual has a macro-organizational perspective, which implies that the individual with the responsibility is more than just an extension of someone with higher status. He is now carrying out an activity which, by its very nature, has its own implicit authority based upon professional or other value-laden standards that are not part of the manager who is assigning the task.

Many managers insist that in delegating work to their subordinates they are assigning a high degree of decision-making authority, when in fact they perceive this as actually establishing an extension of themselves. This confusing message gives a conflicting directive to the subordinate, who is now being held responsible for a task, but who does not have the authority to deliver. In this case, the subordinate is not being delegated to, but is having work assigned to him, which leaves him quite powerless.

The ability to delegate has as its foundation both managerial and human resource skills. In the managerial area, the needed skills are those associated with the traditional and basic functions of management such as planning, organizing, staffing, directing, coordinating, reporting, budgeting, decision making, and controlling. The human resource area is also part of the delegation process, because of the selection and training of those candidates who are considered to be capable of carrying out the assignments. Managers who have a difficult time in assuming this responsibility actually do not know how or what to delegate. Obviously, a surgeon cannot delegate his unique skill during the operation to a subordinate, and a researcher must complete his own research and ultimately write his own reports. Managers can delegate certain aspects of their responsibility in order to unburden themselves for other assignments and endeavors which often have a higher priority. If a manager feels that the decision-making aspects of his position are such that it is necessary for him to do most of the work personally, he may find it difficult to delegate portions of his work to others.

Another set of questions for self-analysis may be helpful at this point to clarify this conflict in managing time:

1. Is there anything that someone else can do better than I can?
2. Am I taking full advantage of the people on my staff who have more knowledge, background, and experience in the work?
3. Is there anything someone else can do at lesser expense than I can?

4. Is there anything someone else can do with better timing than I can?
5. Am I trying to cover too much ground?
6. Is there a proper cut-off point for my personal decisions?

These questions are important because they indicate to the manager what is occurring with regard to his own style, and how well his time is being managed. Or, is his style affecting the effective management of his time? In the majority of cases where a problem exists, we may find that delegation does not actually exist. The solution, of course, is not in the need to hire additional personnel who can execute the tasks of the manager, but in utilizing those human resources available so that they will be able to manage those tasks that are in need of solution.

## THE DELEGATION-PRODUCTIVITY-SATISFACTION LINK

A decline in productivity can be traced to lowered satisfaction because of a failure on the part of the health care manager to delegate. Some suggestions for building delegation into the framework of the organization's philosophy and structure are the following (Lagges, 1979, p. 776):

- structuring the organization to meet long- and short-term objectives
- determining the positions that are required, their scope, and the commensurate authority to perform them
- establishing proper division of responsibility
- defining the role and function of key committees
- ensuring proper span of control
- eliminating excess layers of management
- delineating short and clear lines of communication
- establishing the basis for accountability
- shortening decision channels

Managers must be careful to pass on only those tasks that are their responsibility and to give assignments *only* to their own subordinates. Any attempt to move beyond the scope of their own responsibility could result in duplication of effort and conflicts with other organizational units. Confusion and loss of efficiency can also be minimized by delegating a specific assignment to only one capable individual, rather than requiring responses from several. Duplication of effort resulting from poorly defined job responsibility and ineffectual delegation is a frequent cause of reduced productivity.

# Delegate All

The range of the assigned task also affects efficiency. If possible, it is desirable to entrust responsibility for a complete project or function, rather than assigning only separate duties. Giving an employee full responsibility increases initiative, encourages greater attention to the results, and facilitates the successful completion of the task without unnecessary (and inefficient) coordination with others.

# Delegate Some

However, in some instances, only parts of a project, and not the full assignment, should be assigned. These might include doing basic research, gathering survey data, analyzing costs, conducting interviews, and writing procedures. A primary management responsibility is to delegate the maximum amount of work to the lowest possible level, provided that the work can be done efficiently there. In this and only this way can increased productivity be effected.

# Delegate None

It is obvious, however, that certain functions should not be delegated at all. For example, top management should retain responsibility for strategic planning and board of director issues. Similarly, the responsibility for disciplining and appraising immediate subordinates should not be delegated. An executive who overdelegates is just as inefficient as one who fails to delegate at all (Lagges, 1979, p. 777).

More effective use of executive skill will increase the efficiency of the total organization. Middle-level managers who are given greater responsibility and authority will also benefit. Proper delegation develops the essential skills of subordinates, enriches the job, creates better morale, reduces turnover, and encourages initiative. The organization can benefit because these individuals will be more properly and more quickly prepared for promotion and the assumption of greater responsibility. This saves time.

A study was conducted (Wolf, Breslau, & Novack, 1977, p. 401) to determine the managerial and organizational outcomes of utilizing delegation in primary care teams. The settings for this study were individual and group practices rather than large complex organizations such as hospitals. The variables that were examined were satisfaction, quality, and time. The following findings were extracted from the research:

1. *Satisfaction*—The more the traditional M.D. does himself on a complex problem, the more satisfied he is with work. By contrast, the M.D. in a modern organization finds increasing satisfaction with work as delegation increases on a complex problem.

Similarly, the non-M.D.s in the modern organization tend to experience increasing work, interpersonal, and financial satisfaction as delegation increases.
2. *Quality*—For both M.D.s and non-M.D.s, the results show that in the more traditional organization, as delegation increases perceived quality decreases, while in the modern organization, as delegation increases perceived quality increases within the group practice environment.

## THE FAILURE TO DELEGATE

Many managers are great offenders of the process of delegation. It doesn't matter whether the manager is totally immersed in his work and it is of no consequence that time constraints are being imposed. What is essential is that assignments are being managed by the individual administrator, and he is mistakenly not including subordinates within the sphere of the decision-making process. The unfortunate aspect of this is that subordinates expect to be involved in the decision-making process, since they know that an upward mobility thrust with a managerial position as a target has a prerequisite: the ability to make decisions. Failure to delegate on the part of their supervisor denies them that experience, which leads to frustration and counterproductive stress.

If a manager fails to delegate, it may be important to examine some of the issues that may assist in explaining this phenomenon. These may not be intellectual or cognitive issues, but may be psychological problems that manifest themselves emotionally in dysfunctional behavior. If a manager is aware that he is not performing well with regard to delegation, he must examine certain components of his behavior so that he can understand why he is unable to handle this crucial managerial function. He may wish to examine elements of his personality, experiences, and background to see whether there are any "anchors" keeping him from action, originating from previous or even current behaviors. One major problem, for example, is that some managers have a great fear they will be discovered to be inept. This emotional trauma is quite often debilitating.

Intellectually, the manager often assumes he is performing his job in a satisfactory manner, but at a deeper level his feelings of inadequacy and insecurity are extremely strong and are difficult to handle. He may become immersed in details to overcompensate for these personal shortcomings and therefore be reluctant to delegate from fear that his subordinates and peers will finally see how inept he is. This process, of course, functions at an unconscious level and thus is difficult to recognize. Other managers have an overdeveloped notion of what perfection should be and, therefore, set impossible standards to achieve. A major concern for the frustration level of the manager and his unwillingness to delegate is intertwined in his feelings that he is inadequate in his job and, therefore, he really should not depend upon subordinates who will eventually discover that he is unqualified.

It appears that the higher a manager is in the hierarchy, the more he tends to be oriented to the future with regard to time and planning. By using delegation, this manager would be able to evaluate planning, managing, and assessment activities with regard to their potential for future action. Yet it is not uncommon to find managers who are under stress and pressure engaged in fabricating reasons why subordinates should not be involved in decision making.

Managers also become overwhelmed by "deadline-itis," which creates tension and the feeling that all unfinished assignments and their impending deadlines can only be handled through panic, anxiety, and stress. This has been the traditional conditioning of the manager and is time-consuming and emotionally draining. These managers also attempt to avoid the making of decisions and ensuing delegation by diluting decisions through the vehicle of committees, which is a way of neutralizing the impact of their input. They also do not take full measures to act but only take a partial stand when it is important to focus on a total decision. At the same time, they attempt to delay making decisions by failing to follow up on decisions, so that the major impact of what they should do becomes further diluted. Fatigue is another psychosomatic factor that is responsible for managers not acting upon a decision and allowing them to avoid the necessary process.

It is a common theme that time is an extremely scarce resource and unless it is managed effectively and efficiently nothing else can be managed. Managers who utilize their time effectively have analyzed their personal use of time and have been able to eliminate unproductive demands made upon their time. Most astute managers are cognizant that they do not have unlimited resources and time to perform all aspects of their positions completely, as the time constraints and the complexity of health care operations are ever increasing. One solution to lessening the mounting time pressure is to examine the basic working method and style of the manager, as has been discussed. Another way of improving use of time may be to increase an individual manager's output. As managerial techniques and processes are improved and refined, there should be a commensurate increase in output. When individuals claim they do not have enough time to perform their jobs, this may be a symptom of decreasing output and the accumulating obsolescence of their skills, expertise, and knowledge. This connotes a problem in need of a solution.

## ANXIETY AND PERCEPTION

Managers in health care organizations can increase their output by increasing their capacity to acquire accurate data, based on clear perceptions of what is happening in their domains. To improve their mental "photography," it is recommended that they increase their sensitivity by way of more personal experiences and increased knowledge. This can only occur when they rid themselves of unproductive preoccupation with trivia. If they are capable of altering their routine and acquiring new skills aimed at conserving time, this can be a component of their new streamlined managerial profile. It is important that managers be aware of the fact that at best they can gain only a fraction of the needed data about what is going on. They must check and scan to find out what and how other individuals see events in order to improve the quality of their own perceptions. This can be done by exploring ideas and by being closely in touch with other individuals. Too often managers become overwhelmed by inaccurate perception. As a result of this they spend a great deal of time experiencing anxiety and stress. This state cuts into their productivity by demanding much of their energy in fighting the wrong battle.

Anxiety-ridden managers are usually fearful of not getting credit for a job or fearful that someone else will know more about the job than they do. They have additional fears that their subordinates who are now being given this freedom to decide via delegation will move ahead of them up the organizational ladder while they are left behind. These fears lead to internal and intrapsychic conflicts in which individual supervisors have a most difficult time resolving many of their personal insecurities.

Many of these managers have achieved their positions within the organization as a result of being excellent technicians in their own specialized field. They may not have well-developed skills in imparting information to others, particularly to subordinates. In their own area of expertise they are accustomed to dealing with problems from conception to completion and to using their own resources and skills in isolation. They have discovered that solving problems intuitively is the only safe way to achieve effectiveness and success. To delegate would be a greater personal problem for them, since it would hamper this initial success pattern. A new system with delegation requirements would be uncomfortable for them. One of the prime adjustments managers must make is altering their basic styles from being doers to persons who get things done through other people, which is a basic concept in the classical definition of management. In this case, management and delegation are mutually complementary. Delegation multiplies efforts through the division of duties. It is actually the foundation for organizing, since before anyone can decide how to organize functions and also direct subordinates to perform those tasks, the manager must resolve this conflict that these duties will in fact be done by others and not himself.

In delegation, managers actually give subordinates the right to make decisions, since decision making is the core of both management and delegation. It involves investing trust in subordinates, and lack of trust is largely to blame for initial nondelegation. Delegation is, in certain respects, similar to a personal investment. *The second time a manager delegates to the same subordinate will usually require half the time that the initial delegation process took.* In addition, since ultimate accountability for the subordinate's errors rests with the manager, the manager can actually minimize the chance of mistakes by gradually increasing the challenge of a delegated job. An outstanding performance by a subordinate is a good indicator of an individual's success as a manager and as a delegator. Managers who are being considered for promotion can present the fact that they have capable and trained subordinates to handle their tasks. This allows for upwardly mobile promotion, since a subordinate can step in and take over.

## RAMIFICATIONS OF NONDELEGATION

There are some problems with delegation in which managers and their subordinates fail to agree on the specifics of what is to be delegated (Appelbaum, 1981). Some of these issues include the following situations:

1. Subordinates do not have the necessary training needed in order to complete the delegated tasks. This is a managerial problem that can be overcome by having subordinates fully trained in those aspects of the operation that are essential and for which they will ultimately be held accountable.
2. Managers enjoy their work thoroughly and do not want to delegate the satisfying aspects of their work, delegating only those tasks that are not meaningful or are irrelevant or redundant.
3. Managers will only delegate those assignments with which they are not familiar or at which they are not very proficient. This creates a problem in which managers actually abdicate their role as the controlling force in accountability for a task. When the task is not performed well by the subordinates, the managers can ventilate their frustration and wrath upon the subordinates, which only adds to the basic confusion created by the improper delegation. This in itself becomes a problem that leads to other managerial difficulties. In actuality, when managers face up to unfamiliar or difficult tasks, they actually enhance their versatility at handling broader responsibilities.
4. Another problem is that managers do not usually explain to their subordinates what the overall organizational mission is, and when the subordinates do not understand organizational goals, they have a difficult time in dealing with the delegated responsibilities.
5. Many times managers will choose an overqualified subordinate to assure that the job is being performed properly, which can be traced back to the fact that managers are fearful of mistakes on the part of their subordinates. When they use an overqualified individual, those basic, pedestrian areas of the job that are essential and in need of normal monitoring are often left unmanaged. When managers make it clear to their subordinates that they really mean it when they claim they are completely supporting the process of delegation, then uncompleted or incorrect tasks will not keep coming back as subordinates keep coming in for continuing reassurance and advice.

Delegation is not an all-or-nothing process, but it is a managerial process. This managerial process should be executed through the following steps for managerial initiative. The steps are arranged in a power hierarchy.

1. Subordinate to take action, and no further contact with the manager is necessary.
2. Subordinate to take action, and let the manager know what he did via advice.
3. Subordinate to look into the problem and let the manager know what he intends to do via recommendation and then perform the task unless advised not to.
4. Subordinate to look into the problem and let the manager know what he intends to do: No action to be taken until manager approves.
5. Subordinate to look into the problem and let the manager know alternative actions, enumerate pros and cons of each, and recommend one for approval.
6. Subordinate to look into the problem and report all the facts to the manager, who will decide what to do.

These processes of delegation are the degrees of authority that managers are willing to allow and give to their subordinates. It is essential to understand how they work and when to employ them. It is also necessary to determine at what level the manager is within the organization's decision-making hierarchy and what his own decision-making style is in order to achieve a congruent fit within the complex, dynamic health care environment. The final component of delegation is the necessary follow-up component required of all managers in the form of control.

## CONTROL

One of the best ways to manage the effectiveness of time allocation is by the process of follow up. When a manager intends to delegate to his subordinates, he must be aware that they will be doing the job their own way. This may create a dilemma for the manager if he wants to maintain enough control to avoid problems before he is faced with recurring problems. At one extreme of the continuum are those subordinates who function independently within certain programs and are almost totally free to complete the assignment as they see it. The follow up to this increases degree by degree until the opposite extreme of the continuum is reached in which the authority to utilize all of the data and make the actual decisions is still held completely by the manager.

The amount of control that the manager exercises in the follow up to a delegated task is often determined by the unique personality and style of the manager, the personality and style of his subordinates, and the nature of the task itself. Follow up will most likely be close if the manager has not delegated to the individual previously or when an unknown candidate has been selected to handle a task. When a task has clear precedence, policies, or procedures, less follow up is needed and decisions involving significant departures from any general policy will be held by the manager under careful control. The issues that become difficult are those that remain with the manager after he has delegated the routine decisions of the task to other people. It is important to understand that the managerial functions of leadership, policy making, goal setting, planning, disciplining, and motivating are still in the arena of the manager and even though he delegates, he still is responsible for these aspects. These processes should not be delegated to subordinates and the closer a delegated task comes to one of these prime managerial responsibilities, the more follow up will be required. Follow up also impacts upon the evaluation of a delegated task.

Effective performance is difficult to measure while the individual is performing, and it is essential that when a manager delegates, he follows up at an agreed-upon date when the performance of the task is completed. In discussing exceptional performance it is important for the manager to determine what rewards should follow it. The individual who is successful and has performed all the tasks that have been delegated will appreciate extrinsic rewards as well as those intrinsic rewards gained from having been the recipient of a delegated task. When managers and subordinates both understand the connections among motivation, effort, performance, and intended outcomes, they discover and even internalize the awareness of expectations. If delegation and task accomplishment on the part of subordinates is the manager's expectation, then this communication will be most lucid for both parties. This is one of the most efficient and effective ways of managing responsibility and time as well. The management of time certainly can be connected to the task of delegation since both are inextricably woven together.

One of the methods to be employed by health care organizations seeking a solution to improving time utilization and delegating both responsibility and authority for tasks is the participative process of flextime.

## FLEXTIME—A MODEST UTILIZATION SOLUTION

Flextime (flexible work hours) is a system in which personnel are permitted to choose the hours they wish to work as long as they work a specified number of hours each budget period. There can be flexibility within the work week or work month, and credited time can even be carried forward within specific limits. This allows individuals the freedom to vary their work schedule over a longer period. It also assists the manager in delegating authority and responsibility via participative administration. All health care organizations are under pressure to increase productivity and efficiency at the lowest contained cost. Flextime can be utilized to accomplish this growing need and goal.

## Care Analysis

The Bennett Community Health Center has been utilizing flexible work hours for the past year and a half. The schedule for nine months of the year has established two core time periods each day for the housekeeping department, from 9:30 AM to noon and from 1:30 to 4 PM, during which hours personnel must be present. The core hours are 25 per week and personnel are permitted to establish their own schedules to complete the remaining 15 hours. They can arrange their own time as to when to work, eat lunch, and leave for home. All they owe is the 40 hours per week. This schedule is shown in Figure 3-2.

This case has some interesting ramifications. Research at Hewlett-Packard Corporation (Zawacki & Johnson, 1976, pp. 15-19) revealed that problems do exist with this system, such as managerial resistance to change in any form, including work schedule changes (Stein & Cohen, 1976, pp. 40-43). However, this study did identify some positive features.

As the environment changes, people become more susceptible to messages that help them to restructure the situation. The introduction of flextime into an organization can have unsettling effects for the managers' environment. They often feel that they will have to deal with a new, bewildering set of problems. To overcome this mental state, at Hewlett-Packard the ground rules and the policies for handling vacations, holidays, and absences, as well as the procedures for dealing with specific problems relating to abuse of the system, were formalized in writing. This formalization had the effect of providing a new structure and set of norms that the managers could adopt, which gave them a sense of comfort and structure.

Several studies have shown that a surprising number of managers at all levels of the organization have very risk-aversive behavior and if they perceive flextime as a potential risk, they will be likely to resist it. One of the most effective means of reducing the perceived risk is to establish the program on a trial basis for a few months. In fact, at Hewlett-Packard a trial approach was used for subsequent implementations, even though the early programs had demonstrated no major problems. The trial provides a psychological "escape valve" and reduces the level of perceived risk (Morgan, 1977, p. 96).

Since no system is perfect, flexible work hours have both assets and liabilities. Some of these are discussed here.

## Advantages for Management

1. Most managers who utilize flexible work hours appear to feel that the employees have developed a more responsible attitude toward their work. Jobs in hand tend to be finished, and team spirit is encouraged where individuals have to consult each other before making a group decision about

**Figure 3-2** Bennett Community Health Center—Flexible Work Hours Schedule (Housekeeping)

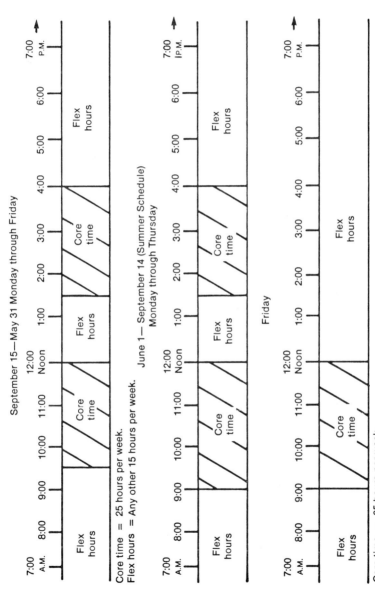

September 15—May 31 Monday through Friday

Core time = 25 hours per week.
Flex hours = Any other 15 hours per week.

June 1— September 14 (Summer Schedule)
Monday through Thursday

Friday

Core time = 25 hours per week.
Flex hours = Any other 15 hours per week.

starting and finishing times. Flextime has eliminated excuses for lateness or absences from work on personal business.

2. Work performance seems to be more efficient due to the reduction in the number of days lost through *alleged* illness and to the reduction in cost for a given output; these results are due to a more highly motivated work force and the need for less overtime. (The usual gossip at the beginning and end of each day tends to be reduced, with employees arriving in a random manner and settling quietly down to work.) Furthermore, the system has created a quiet time—that is, the periods outside core time—when output can be more effective due to fewer interruptions.

3. There may be organizational improvements. For example, communications may improve, since more precise instructions to subordinates tend to be necessary. Also, the capital assets of a firm may be better used because of the larger total work period each day.

4. Flextime can be seen as a labor attraction. A reduction in labor turnover is likely because employees who are accustomed to a flexible system are less likely to be attracted to organizations that do not offer such a system. This appeal could lead to a reduction in recruitment and training costs.

5. Flextime can increase employee commitment. Basically, people want to work; when working conditions are right, employees willingly cooperate with management. Trust placed in a company's employees is repaid. Virtually all organizations operating on flexible working hours claim that the working climate has been improved. Employees no longer see themselves as nine-to-fivers, but as responsible human beings; their commitment is increased and the organization benefits as a result (Butteriss & Albrecht, 1979, p. 52).

## Disadvantages for Management

1. Additional costs may arise from the need for time-recording equipment; no matter which system is adopted, some cost is incurred.

2. Administrative costs increase, but they can be controlled by leaving a good deal of paperwork to the employees themselves.

3. Overhead may increase as an office or factory will have to be open longer; heating, lighting, and other such expenses will rise.

4. There may be some operational inconvenience because employees are not always present when required. Supervisory difficulties may occur, and additional supervisors may be required to cover the extra time bands. Communications may deteriorate as the fixed time when employees are obliged to be available is reduced, in some cases to four hours a day.

5. The problem of assuring safety and security also arises. A British company found that it would have safety problems in its laboratory; its flexible time is

therefore limited, since no one is allowed to carry out work of a dangerous nature alone in the laboratory.

6. There may also be miscellaneous disadvantages. Some workers may deliberately build up credit time by "staying over" for longer than the job demands. Friction may sometimes develop between employees who have the freedom of a flexible system and those who are excluded or restricted because of the job they do (Butteriss & Albrecht, 1979, p. 55).

## Advantages for the Employees

1. Flextime allows employees to work according to their personal rhythms; some people are at their best first thing in the morning, while others are happier working later in the afternoon or in the evening. This flexibility tends to reduce the stress and strain of having to work fixed hours at predetermined times.
2. There is a better balance between private life and work. An individual has more opportunity to plan his or her free time and private life. People have more time for their families and their private time is much fuller and more satisfying.
3. Travelling to and from work can be far less exhausting and harrowing as the rush hours can be avoided; the employee can arrive at work feeling much more relaxed. If a large number of workers in a large city begin to work on flextime schedules, the overall intensity of the rush-hour traffic will certainly decrease; traffic accident rates may also decline. Trends such as flextime may eventually lead to the elimination of the traditional weekend, which would improve enormously the utilization of public resources and recreation facilities.
4. In many systems, the employee can amass credit hours, and the company may allow him to take a half-day or a whole day off in lieu. This advantage is clearly seen. However, it must once again be emphasized that time off during core time will be given only after consultation with the department head.
5. There are also economic advantages: travelling expenses may decrease by travelling at off-peak times; lateness and financial penalties disappear and many employees, through the nature of their jobs, have always expected to work additional time where necessary without extra pay. With flextime this additional time is credited (Butteriss & Albrecht, 1979, p. 54).

## Disadvantages for the Employees

1. There may be some economic disadvantages. Overtime may be reduced because of more effective output. Productivity may rise, but employees may not share the benefits of the increase. In some cases, personal absence privileges, such as for medical visits, may be lost.

2. The introduction of flextime may also have some adverse effects on working conditions. For example, the necessity for time recording may be regarded as a decrease in status or another form of management control. The level of supervision may fall at the extremes of the day, and some employees may find that it is not available when required.

The advantages and disadvantages of flexible work hours have been clearly identified for the manager to utilize as a decision-making guide. It seems clear that the ramifications of any decision in this area must be carefully considered before any action is taken.

Time management strategies raise several important questions for managers of organizations:

- If someone uses time management and actually gets more done in less time, should he be rewarded?

- Are there enough job duties to warrant an official time management program, since they do take time, effort and money?

- What are the advantages (and disadvantages) of knowing your job so well thanks to the self-analysis techniques?

- Do managers really want to delegate, or will this be seen as a loss of power?

There are doubtless more questions of equal importance. The crucial thing is that these issues be addressed when considering the use of time management. Time management means less stress for individuals, which means more efficient, satisfied, healthy employees, which in turn means more effective organizations (Schuler, 1979, p. 854). This effectiveness in reducing conflict, improving delegation, and time efficiency is a viable goal of the health care organization.

---

**REFERENCES**

Appelbaum, S.H. *Stress management for health care providers*. Rockville, Md.: Aspen Systems, 1981.

Bonoma, T.V., & Slevin, D.P. *Executive survival manual*. Boston: CBI Publishing Co., 1978.

Butteriss, M., & Albrecht, K. *New management tools*. Englewood Cliffs, N.J.: Prentice-Hall, 1979.

Drucker, P.F. How to manage your time. *Harper's Magazine*, December 1966, 56.

Drucker, P.F. *The effective executive*. New York: Harper and Row, 1967.

Dunnette, M.D. (Ed.). *Handbook of Industrial and Organizational Psychology*, "Communication in Organizations" by L. Porter & K. Roberts. Chicago: Rand McNally Co., 1976.

Jackson, J.H., & Hayen, R.L. Rationing the scarcest resource: A manager's time. *Personnel Journal*, October 1974, *53*(10), 753-755.

Lagges, J.G. The role of delegation in improving productivity. *Personnel Journal,* November 1979, *58*(11), 776.

McConkey, D. *No nonsense delegation.* New York: American Management Association, 1974.

Morgan, F.T. Your (flex) time may come. *Personnel Journal,* February 1977, *56*(2), 96.

Schuler, R.S. Managing stress means managing time. *Personnel Journal,* December 1979, *58*(12), 854.

Stein, B., & Cohen, A. Flextime, work when you want to. *Psychology Today,* June 1976, *10,* 40-43.

Wolf, G., Breslau, N., & Novack, A. The effect of delegation on outcomes in the primary care team. *Proceedings of the Academy of Management, 37th Annual Meeting,* 1977, 401.

Zawacki, R.A., & Johnson, J.S. Alternate workweek schedules—one company's experience with flextime. *Supervisory Management,* June 1976, *21,* 15-19.

# Chapter 4

# Planning for Time and Direction

TIME MANAGEMENT HIGHLIGHTS

1. Consistently waiting until the last minute or delaying to plan or take action until an emergency exists forces decisions to be made under crisis conditions, which compresses time.
2. The strength of a good health care manager lies in his ability to make the right decisions and to ask the right questions where there is an absence of understanding.
3. Planning for time and direction is a process of determining how the organization can get to where it wants to go and what exactly it will do to accomplish its goals.
4. One of the planning models employed in health care is the decision matrix, which is a management technique needed to help allocate time priorities and related evaluations.
5. Another model to consider is the Gantt Chart, which is a management technique to initially plan for and monitor working time as a control mechanism. It provides an overall visible means for setting goals and scheduling time use in order to attain those goals. It also permits observations of accomplishments and a more effective reassignment of time to handle unexpected contingencies and demands.
6. Program Evaluation and Review Technique (PERT) is another technique to furnish time estimates. This process requires the setting of objectives and designating sequences of events to attain goals.
7. The systems approach is also used by the administrator to evaluate existing conditions, change and improve the current state of the process, and finally, to design something new for the process to

stimulate performance to an optimum level. This approach possesses four basic steps: problem formulation, modeling, analysis-
optimization, and implementation.
8. Systems can be classified as being:
   a. linear or nonlinear
   b. continuous or discrete
   c. constant or time varying
   d. lumped or distributed
   e. probabilistic or deterministic
9. Gaming is another decision-making technique to deal with complexity by permitting reality-oriented interaction to occur within a
   simulated health care environment to save time lost because of poor
   planning. PPBS systems also accomplish this.
10. Strategic planning is becoming an essential tool of the health care
    manager since it is a continuous process of making present entre-
    preneurial (risk-taking) decisions systematically and with the great-
    est knowledge of their futurity; organizing systematically the efforts
    needed to carry out these decisions; and measuring the results of
    these decisions against the expectations through organized, sys-
    tematic feedback. It is a means used to achieve the ends (objectives)
    via a comprehensive major plan. This is usually accomplished in
    hospitals by the chief administrator with the cooperation of the
    board and medical staff.

Each new workday brings another set of situations and contingencies in need of
management. While many of the resulting demands on available time are quite
normal and routine, sometimes—and sometimes it seems too often—the unexpected happens. These unannounced surprises, which can strike swiftly and
devastatingly, may be highly disconcerting and diversionary, forcing the aban-
donment of existing plans and requiring immediate action. In an emergency the
usual course of events is abruptly interrupted and replaced either by a step-by-step
predetermined plan or by an attempt to implement solutions on a trial and error
basis, often accompanied by considerable confusion, expense, and wasted time.
    A classic example of an unexpected emergency was the now famous power
blackout that struck New York City in 1965 during the evening rush hour. So many
things were dependent upon electricity—subways, elevators, traffic lights, street
lights, and residential lighting—that the city came to a screeching halt. Many
people hitchhiked or walked long hours to reach their homes, while others never
made it back, spending the night in public buildings or other places of refuge.
    Another kind of emergency can develop within an organization itself, and is not
the result of an external shock or disaster. Rather, in this situation someone fails to
take proper action at the proper time, due either to lapse of memory or just ordinary

procrastination. Whatever the reason, delaying or neglecting to implement a necessary action makes a bad condition worse, as for example, in delaying roof repairs until both costs and safety factors are compounded. These situations can usually be avoided, or at least controlled, by the exercise of some informal planning or foresight.

Consistently waiting to plan or take action until an emergency arises forces decisions to be made under crisis conditions, which often precludes the opportunity to evaluate all available options. In addition, as time is stolen from other activities, other potential crises are spawned. People who work in such unstable environments usually consider themselves firefighters, continually battling the neverending progression of emergency situations through crisis management.

At the other extreme are occasions when events operate exactly oppositely to a crisis. In these situations activities may be intentionally prolonged to fill the available time. This is the phenomenon known as Parkinson's Law: "Work expands so as to fill the time available for its completion" (Parkinson, 1957, p. 2). Compared to the feverish pitch of activity in an emergency, in these instances work proceeds slowly and discretionary time exists for a wide variety of other interests and activities.

## THE NEED FOR SETTING PRIORITIES

It is frequently desirable and necessary to assign priorities for the use of one's time somewhere in between these two extremes. To aid in this process, some questions can be asked at this juncture:

- How can you decide what job should be started and completed first?

- Is the one that is most time-consuming the one to begin first, or should it be left for later?

- What is really most important and what least important?

- How can you best allocate your time to satisfy both your needs and the needs of an organization?

The strength of a good manager lies in his ability to make the right decisions and to ask the right questions. It is interesting to note, however, that most managers view their supervisory task as mainly consisting of answering the queries of subordinates. On the contrary, the art of managing requires question-asking skills that need continual practice on the part of the manager if he is to be an effective problem solver (Bennett, 1978, p. 194). Asking the right questions can also save great amounts of time. Table 4-1 indicates some of the questions that need to be asked.

**Table 4-1** Questions for Managers

| Dimension | Question | Comment |
|-----------|----------|---------|
| 1. Purpose | What is being done? Why is it being done? What else might be done? | The answers to these questions help to eliminate unnecessary parts of the job. |
| 2. Place | Where is it being done? Why is it done there? Does it need to be done at that particular place? Where else might it be done? | |
| 3. Sequence | When is it done? Why is it done then? Does it need to be done at that particular time? When might it be done? | The answers to questions 2, 3, and 4 often suggest that parts of the job can be combined or the sequence, place, or person can be changed. |
| 4. Person | Who is doing it? Why does that person do it? Could it be done better by someone else? Who else might do it? | |
| 5. Means | How is it being done? Why is it done this way? How else might it be done? | These questions are asked with a view toward improving or simplifying the necessary details of the job. |

*Source:* Bennett, 1978, p. 195.

Deciding how to utilize time is a troublesome and unpleasant chore for some people, and something to be avoided. These individuals may prefer to have the decision made for them. Others, however, are willing and anxious to make such decisions and derive satisfaction from setting goals and then planning how to use time to achieve the desired objectives. This can take place quite informally or even without any conscious effort. In a highly structured environment, however, planning may be a rather formal procedure involving discussions between a superior and subordinate. Ideally, mutual agreement should be reached on one or more viable objectives which, within a specified time period, will further the goals of the organization and at the same time provide a sense of fulfillment for the individual. This process also forms the basis for allocating time priorities to perform the stated duties of a job while achieving the agreed-upon objective.

Planning is now a major component of the health care environment. In essence, planning is the process of determining how the organization can get where it wants to go and what exactly the organization will do to accomplish its goals. The changing role of the professional nurse is a case in point. Nurses are becoming more involved in planning and organizing health care activities and are also becoming more responsible for managing and delivering total patient care services. In this new role, managerial responsibilities often include the supervision of other nursing and ancillary personnel, as well as the accomplishment of a wide range of organizational, patient care, and personal objectives.

For efficient allocation of time and effort in working toward these interrelated objectives, the supervisory nurse must decide which objectives are most important, which problems are most critical in impeding goal accomplishment, and how to solve these problems for best results. This task is not always easy because of the possible conflicts existing among the various objectives—for example, the delivery of quality patient care conflicting with the hospital's objective of reducing costs.

Similarly, some methods of solving a problem may help in accomplishing one objective but hinder the accomplishment of another. Initiating a procedure that requires more reporting of patient care information may increase the coordination of unit activities, but decrease the amount of time each nurse may spend actually delivering care to patients. Thus, the nursing supervisor's role requires continual tradeoffs in allocating time and effort toward solving problems—the kind of role conflict that may create stress (Dittrich, Lang, & White, 1979, p. 314).

Some planning models will be explored which are intended to improve the effectiveness, efficiency, and time management skills of the health care professional.

## DECISION MATRIX

A management technique that is helpful in allocating time priorities and related evaluations is called the decision matrix. This basic device applies the idea of expected value as a means of appraising alternate opportunities where outcomes are considered otherwise doubtful or uncertain. The first step, of course, is to determine the particular duties and responsibilities of a specific job. A good place to start is with the job description, which briefly spells out what is to be done. The next step is to make a list of objectives that are both desirable and feasible. Tables 4-2 and 4-3 contain listings of possible duties and objectives for two hypothetical jobs—one in a personnel department and one in an electronic data processing unit.

**Table 4-2** Partial Listing of Duties and Objectives for an Administrative Position in a Personnel Department

| Duties | Objectives |
|---|---|
| Recruit employees | Reduce employee turnover |
| Interview candidates | Reduce absenteeism |
| Select employees | Revise reporting forms |
| Conduct training programs | Provide better informa- |
| Assign employees | tion to employees |
| Prepare reports | Develop new training |
| Administrate pension and | module |
| welfare fund programs | Improve interpersonal |
| Counsel employees | relations |
| Participate in union | Develop new sources of |
| procedures | employees |
| Establish job and wage | Improve filing procedures |
| standards | |

**Table 4-3** Partial Listing of Duties and Objectives for an Administrative Position in an Electronic Data Processing Unit

| Duties | Objectives |
|---|---|
| Maintain | Improve communication |
| Medical records | with other departments |
| Inventory records | Meet report deadlines |
| Payroll records | Eliminate redundant |
| Accounts payable | reports |
| Accounts receivable | Develop new program for |
| Issue payroll checks | pharmacy inventory |
| Issue vendor checks | control |
| Train new personnel | Secure new sources of |
| Provide recurring reports | personnel |
| Provide nonrecurring | Revise reporting forms |
| reports | |

Table 4-4 is a Decision Matrix Chart designed for setting time priorities for a purchasing manager in a health care institution. Because of the constraint of space, only four duties are ranked as column headings across the top of the chart. Similarly, only five objectives are listed along the left margin. It should be noted that both duties and objectives need not be limited to just a few as indicated, but rather should be selected in accordance with individual needs and later reviewed and revised as required.

**Table 4-4** Decision Matrix Chart: Method for Establishing Priorities for Distributing Time in Relation to Job Objectives and Performance of Specified Duties

| OBJECTIVES | (1) Factor | (2) Shop market | | DUTIES (3) Have goods available when needed | | (4) Prepare reports | | (5) Train subordinates | |
|---|---|---|---|---|---|---|---|---|---|
| | | Wgt. | Value | W | V | W | V | W | V |
| Secure lowest price consistent with quality | 20 | .30 | 6.0 | .30 | 6.0 | .10 | 2.0 | .10 | 2.0 |
| Improve vendor relations | 15 | .40 | 6.0 | .20 | 3.0 | .20 | 3.0 | .30 | 4.5 |
| Discover new sources | 20 | .40 | 8.0 | 0 | 0 | 0 | 0 | 0 | 0 |
| Reduce shrinkage | 20 | .20 | 4.0 | .30 | 6.0 | .30 | 6.0 | .10 | 2.0 |
| Reduce value of inventory | 25 | .40 | 10.0 | .40 | 10.0 | .40 | 10.0 | .40 | 10.0 |
| Weighted totals | | | 34.0 | | 25.0 | | 21.0 | | 18.5 |
| Probability | | | .80 | | .95 | | .80 | | .90 |
| Final evaluation | | | 27.20 | | 23.75 | | 16.80 | | 16.65 |

Column 1 is headed by the word "factor," and in the spaces of this column, to the right of each objective, the decision maker should enter a number chosen from 0 to 100 to reflect the relative importance of each objective, compared to all the objectives that are listed. A value of 30, for example, indicates double the significance of 15, and a 0 means no value at all. In the chart, the objective "Reduce Value of Inventory" is rated high with a 25, compared to "Improve Vendor Relations," which only carries a 15. Each of the vertical duty columns is split into two parts. The left side allows for entering a numerical weight or percentage that estimates the chance or probability of attaining each objective as each duty is performed. A similar value from 0 to 100 is recorded in the "Weight" column for each duty/objective combination. This number is, of course, a completely subjective percentage estimate based on individual judgment and experience.

Referring again to the chart, it is estimated there is a 30 out of 100 percent chance to "Improve Vendor Relations" while performing the duty of "Train Subordinates." On the other hand, the probability to "Reduce Value of Inventory" through "Shop Market" is set at 40 percent. After all the weights have been entered, the next step merely requires multiplying the factor figure by each assigned weight and entering the product in the appropriate space of the value columns for all objective/duty combinations. The next procedure is to total each value column in order to determine "Weighted Totals" at the bottom of the chart. A final computation involves estimating the probability of actually fulfilling the responsibility of each duty. When the "Weighted Totals" are multiplied by these last probabilities, the results are entered on the "Final Evaluation" bottom line of the chart. In the example, "Shop Market" earned the highest final total, while "Train Subordinates," the lowest. The duties are then ranked in numerical order, with the one generating the highest "Final Evaluation" (expected value) deserving of the most time and attention. A point to consider is that percentages need not total 100, as each evaluation is considered independent of each other.

While this example is perhaps oversimplified, it does provide a framework for easily developing many kinds of probability estimates or expected values for various duty/objective mixes. As such, it should go far as a handy tool to assist in discovering and assigning priorities, and thus in deciding on direction and time allocation.

The decision matrix is only as good as the information and judgment of those using the chart. It is most effective under conditions of uncertainty and as a technique to help sort out rankings among a number of interacting variables. It is one way of forcing evaluation for the purpose of establishing time priorities. No guarantee of success can be claimed, due to constraints and changing conditions over which there is little control. It is, of course, mandatory to correctly identify and select those duties and objectives to be appraised in order to make the best possible decision. There may be times when peripheral issues arise and become exaggerated, so that the original decision is obscured by unimportant details or distortions. The crux of the decision can, however, be reestablished by raising questions such as: Why? For what purpose? What is to be done? Is that part of this job?

Once priorities have been established, they should not be considered immutable, but should be subject to frequent reevaluation in accordance with changing exogenous and endogenous variables. The main reason for using this type of decision matrix is to help find solutions for better use of available time that meet both the needs of the individual and the goals of the health care institution. In management terms this should go far to maximize benefits and minimize losses.

The key to getting work done properly and on time is quite basic—managers must plan ahead, and then link that plan to a carefully established time schedule. This can work almost as well for individual use as for managing a hospital, a railroad, or an airline. The initial step, of course, is to decide what has to be done and then, by using a decision matrix, determine a ranking of priorities. Next, a practical strategy of attack must be developed, and finally, a time frame must be established within which the work is to be completed. Because of unforeseen difficulties, emergencies, and surprises, which invariably erupt at the least expected and most inconvenient times, it is useful to build in cushions of time (contingencies) that allow for some latitude for alternate courses of action, for example, a hospital could plan to use backup generators in case of a power blackout.

## THE GANTT CHART

This management technique can be applied as a control mechanism to initially plan and then monitor work time. As an added feature, it also provides an early warning system when slippage occurs, indicating what and how much additional time is or can possibly be made available. This concept, originally developed during the early 1900s by Henry Gantt (1919), a pioneer in the field of management, was designed for scheduling factory production runs. While it is still used for that purpose today, it is also particularly applicable to the management of time within health care organizations.

In brief, a Gantt Chart allows observation and evaluation of progress toward the completion of established objectives as measured against a previously determined time schedule. Actually, this is something like setting up a realistic budget and then comparing actual expenditures, in this case time instead of money, with what was previously planned.

Table 4-5 is a simplified version of a Gantt Chart which illustrates only the major duties for a person in charge of a materials management department. The inevitable and numerous office routines are omitted. A brief explanation may generate interest and encouragement in using the chart as a means of planning and controlling what you want to do when it has to be done. In this illustration, the chart highlights an eight-hour, five-day work week plus the first three days of the succeeding week. The planned and expected duties and activities are listed vertically along the left margin of the diagram. The days of the week are indicated across the top of the chart.

**Table 4-5** Gantt Chart

Work Planned [

Work Completed ——

Week 1:

| ACTIVITY | MONDAY | TUESDAY | WEDNESDAY | THURSDAY | FRIDAY |
|---|---|---|---|---|---|
| Inventory review | [ | | | | |
| Interview salesman | | | | [ | |
| Negotiate contract "A" | | [ | [ | | |
| Discuss specs with engineering | | | | | |
| Write report | [ | | | | |
| Attend convention | | | | | [ |
| Interview job applicants | | | | | |
| Prepare budget | | | | | |

Week 2:

| ACTIVITY | MONDAY | TUESDAY | WEDNESDAY |
|---|---|---|---|
| Inventory review | | H | |
| Interview salesman | [ | O | [ |
| Negotiate contract "A" | | L | |
| Discuss specs with engineering | | I | |
| Write report | | D | |
| Attend convention | | A | |
| Interview job applicants | [ | Y | |
| Prepare budget | | | |

The symbols on the chart which resemble a staple, or a ⌐‾‾‾⌐ , are used to indicate the time planned to perform each major job duty or activity. Solid lines directly below show how much of the task was actually accomplished during the specified time period. For example, the job "write report" was planned for Tuesday morning, with the afternoon set aside for a meeting to "negotiate contract A." As it turned out, however, the report was not finished Tuesday morning (indicated by a shortened solid line underneath the "work planned" symbol), and further work on it had to be postponed because of the negotiating meeting scheduled for the afternoon. The short "work completed" line for Tuesday afternoon demonstrates that discussions about contract A were not finished either, and so, for that day, two planned objectives remain to be completed. Due to the interest in concluding contract negotiations as quickly as possible, another meeting was immediately scheduled for Thursday afternoon, in a time slot which previously was deliberately left free to accommodate an unexpected delay or pressing problem.

Another difficulty still remains, however—the report for presentation at the convention scheduled for all day Friday is also not finished, and so now, on Thursday morning, some time decisions must be made. A number of options do exist and are worth exploring. One quick solution would be to complete the report later tonight either at the office or at home. (Hopefully this would not interfere with any personal commitment.) Another would be to have someone else "interview job applicants" or attend the afternoon contract talks. Finally, either the job interviews or the negotiations could be postponed to the latter part of next week. Actually, what should happen in this hypothetical case is that the manager should make an immediate assessment of the situation and do the most urgent activity first, given the limits of his time.

The advantages of using a Gantt Chart as a technique for planning, scheduling, and controlling are readily apparent. It is unique in that it provides an overall visible means for setting goals and then scheduling time use in order to attain those goals. In addition, it permits observations of accomplishments and a more effective reassignment of time to take care of unexpected contingencies and demands. A Gantt Chart is also helpful in situations where an unexpected delay causes a period of unplanned waiting time. An inspection of the chart shows possible readjustments to fill the time vacuum created by being trapped in an unexpected holding pattern. If a meeting is cancelled, be sure some alternate activity can be readily implemented as a backup task to save that precious resource—time.

The opportunity to conveniently shift time allocations and to reorder priorities can help identify the immediately required time in periods of severe time constraints, while still preserving possible alternatives to fulfill previously planned objectives. For the "firefighters" who must respond to emergency situations, the Gantt Chart is a means of refocusing attention and effort once the brush fire has been extinguished. It thus becomes an adjustable timetable for rescheduling time priorities to fulfill objectives.

Table 4-6 lists a few suggestions that should prove useful in devising and implementing your own Gantt Chart.

One final note: Some people in attempting to cope with a difficult problem may see or consider only one alternate solution or option. The Gantt Chart visibly displays an individual's entire time schedule, showing sequences and interdependencies of events and activities, and thus permits a broader view; it should therefore help in seeking and finding the most desirable of a number of possible solutions.

## PROGRAM EVALUATION REVIEW TECHNIQUE (PERT)

PERT as a management technique evolved from the basic concepts contained in the Gantt Chart. The idea was originated in the late 1950s by the Dupont Company as the Critical Path Method (CPM). When the U.S. Navy developed the Polaris Missile System, it devised, with the consulting assistance of Booz, Allen and Hamilton, Inc. and the Lockheed Missile Systems Division, a somewhat similar procedure designated as Program Evaluation and Review Technique (PERT). This technique utilized statistical probability theory to furnish three-time estimates

---

**Table 4-6** Checklist for Using a Gantt Chart for Time Management

1. Consider the Gantt Chart as a budget—plan your time carefully.
2. Be realistic and practical about using your time. Plan what is possible.
3. List only major time-consuming events, activities, and duties of a recurring and nonrecurring nature.
4. Plan and schedule on at least a weekly basis.
5. Build in occasional discretionary time for surprises and emergencies.
6. Have backup activities for unexpected vacuums.
7. If necessary, use reserves of time—hours in excess of a normal work period.
8. Plan changes of pace and subject matter.
9. Give yourself *short* breaks for reflection and relaxation.
10. Set time limits for the duration of meetings, interviews, lunches, visits, and telephone calls.
11. Plan for interruptions when activities exceed time limitations.
12. When required, be unreachable—allow no interruptions by spending day at home, having a "do not disturb sign" at office, or not taking telephone calls.
13. Under duress, delegate—send a surrogate to meetings or to perform a specific duty.
14. Be flexible; reschedule time when and if possible.
15. Evaluate and review your performance on a daily basis.
16. Keep on schedule.
17. Be wary of nibblers—people who frequently ask for "a minute" and take ten—or more.

(pessimistic, most probable, and optimistic) and added events to the graphing of activities (Archibald & Villoria, 1967, pp. 12-15). Taken together, the network techniques of PERT and CPM served to plan a network of activities, their relationships, and their interaction along a path to a given completion date. This graph of paths keeps managerial attention on the project (Wren, 1972, p. 479). Perhaps PERT or CPM is best known for its use in connection with large and complicated projects such as building skyscrapers, ocean liners, or hydroelectric dams. PERT also has applications for much less complex activities, however, particularly in time management because it, like a Gantt Chart, is based on the use of resources to accomplish stated objectives within established time constraints. It is adaptable to use by small groups of people or even individuals when time is a significant element in the attainment of goals. Briefly, the PERT concept requires:

- setting of objectives,
- designating sequences of events or activities to attain goals,
- organizing and coordinating people, materials, and equipment,
- exercising control over the progress of the entire project to ensure completion as scheduled.

It is a planning, scheduling, organizing, coordinating, and controlling technique.

PERT, as a management technique, makes a number of important assumptions which form the basis for its successful adoption:

1. Some activities must occur or be completed before others can start. Before putting a roof on a new facility, the walls must be in place.
2. Some activities take longer to accomplish than others and therefore should start sooner. It may take longer to get delivery of an EKG system than operating room equipment.
3. Some activities can occur concurrently. Doors and windows can be installed at the same time.
4. It is possible to reallocate or reassign some resources from one activity to another in order to avoid postponing the projected completion date. One worker can be sent to pick up needed supplies rather than waiting for a delivery next week.

Figure 4-1 is a representation of a PERT network which was prepared for planning a recognition banquet for health care personnel with ten years of service. Customarily a PERT diagram is read from left to right. In this example each step in the process is indicated by the circled letters, A through I. A first thing to do, quite logically, is to announce the start of the project. Once that is accomplished, a

**Figure 4-1** Program Evaluation and Review Technique

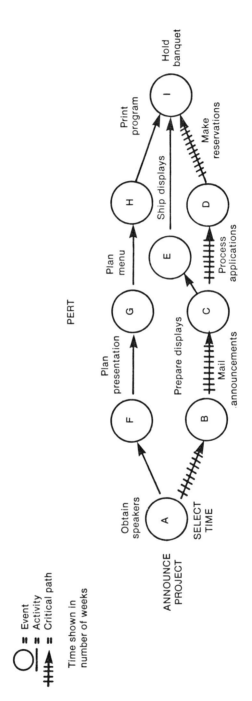

Planning a Banquet

number of other separate sequential tasks can be planned—as shown by the three tracks, A-B-C-D-I, C-E-I, and A-F-G-H-I. The numbers that appear between the lettered steps represent the estimated time it will take to complete each separate task along that particular track. For example, the number 2 between A and B means that 2 weeks are allocated for selecting a time and site from the starting date of the project. Mailing announcements should be completed in 3 weeks, in moving along from B to C. Because the track A through I takes 12 weeks and thus more time than A-F-G-H-I (10 weeks), or A-B-C-E-I (8 weeks), it is called the "critical path." Any delay along this longest track will cause a postponement of the banquet, (I). For instance, assuming the estimated times as being accurate, if the announcements are sent out the fourth, rather than the third week, the whole project will be delayed one week. Thus, in order to keep on schedule, the announcements must be mailed during the third week. As noted above, A-F-G-H-I requires only 10 weeks and therefore two extra weeks, called slack, are available along this track. This means the activities along this route or network can be delayed by as much as two weeks without affecting the date originally set for the banquet. Similarly H, which is scheduled for the seventh week, need not begin until the ninth week. The flexibility or rescheduling capability for this PERT is shown on Table 4-7. By subtracting the "latest start time" from the "scheduled time," the amount of slack time is determined. Figure 4-2 is a variance of PERT using a systems approach to chart organizational activities through the medium of time.

One other important aspect of PERT should be mentioned. In the event that a blockage causes a delay along the critical path, or for that matter any other track, it is not necessary to accept the condition and announce a new later completion date,

---

**Table 4-7** PERT Activity Chart

| | Activity | Scheduled time | | Latest time | | Slack |
|---|---|---|---|---|---|---|
| | | Start | End | Start | End | time |
| A-B | Select sites | 0 | 2 | 0 | 2 | 0 |
| B-C | Mail announcements | 2 | 5 | 2 | 5 | 0 |
| C-D | Process applications | 5 | 10 | 5 | 10 | 0 |
| D-I | Make reservations | 10 | 12 | 10 | 12 | 0 |
| A-F | Obtain speakers | 0 | 2 | 2 | 4 | 2 |
| F-G | Plan special presentation | 2 | 4 | 4 | 6 | 2 |
| G-H | Plan menu | 4 | 7 | 6 | 9 | 2 |
| H-I | Print program | 7 | 10 | 9 | 12 | 2 |
| C-E | Prepare displays | 5 | 6 | 9 | 10 | 4 |
| E-I | Ship displays | 6 | 8 | 10 | 12 | 4 |

**Figure 4-2** Diagramming Organizational Activities via Time

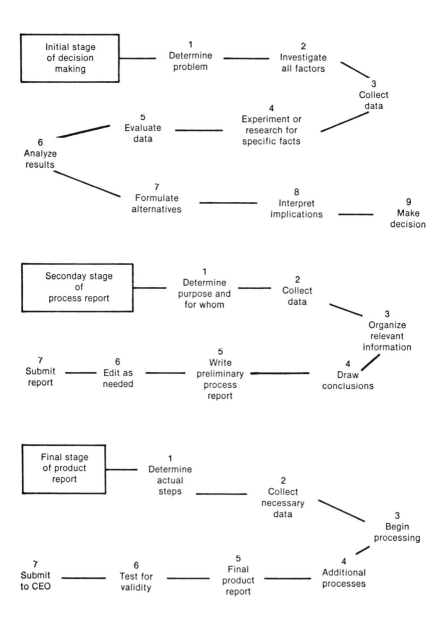

or go into a crisis situation by attempting to adhere to the original schedule and hiring new resources or authorizing double or triple overtime pay. It may be quite possible to transfer or shift existing resources from a network having slack to the one experiencing difficulty. This procedure assumes that the resources are mobile and capable of performing the required functions. This kind of action includes moving people or equipment or both.

Where a PERT system is developed with a great many long-range and sophisticated networks, probability theory is used for estimating the chance of achieving specific completion dates and the entire plan is computerized.

To summarize, the following benefits accrue from using a PERT as a time management tool:

- Provides logical and visible sequences of activities.

- Schedules activities in accordance with a predetermined completion date.

- Communicates the present status of a project and thus allows for evaluation and necessary remedial actions.

- Indicates the existence of available slack time, which allows shifting rather than employing additional resources.

- Allows for the coordination and integration of a number of activities toward attaining a common objective.

- Pinpoints responsibility and problems.

Finally, a few caveats are worth noting:

- A PERT does not guarantee that either the individual activities or the entire project will be completed as planned. This technique is subject to many uncontrollable variables, including the unpredictable vagaries of human beings.

- The available resources may not be adaptable or transferable because of the need to hold costs to a minimum while maintaining the original schedule.

- Any plan is only as good as the ability of the person or persons who devise it. It is based on human judgment and, therefore, is subject to human error.

A PERT network will perform the basic management functions of planning, organizing, staffing, coordinating, and controlling and will result in the more effective use of time. Another concept that can aid the health care manager in time management is the systems approach, which is especially applicable since a system is an intended collection of interacting entities—which describes the hospital quite well.

## SYSTEMS APPROACH TO HEALTH CARE AND TIME MANAGEMENT

Systems activity is concerned with the review, evaluation, and improvement of the methods and procedures by which input units of work are processed so as to produce a satisfactory output. There are a number of opportunities available to the health care manager for developing changes in systems activity that will provide more effective and efficient ways of processing work in the work unit.

When the department manager is faced with the demands for results that confront today's hospital, he will most often experience constraints in terms of the quantity and quality of resources available to him. Therefore, the manager must actively look for and find new methods that will ensure effective and efficient use of resources. The department manager cannot continue to produce the same output over time, because it is reasonable to expect that the users of that output will demand new and better outcomes from the manager's functional unit. This healthy dissatisfaction that keeps change for improvement in the forefront is the very ingredient that moves the organization forward to higher levels of achievement (Bennett, 1978, p. 149).

In the management of a health care organization, the systems approach is often applied to complex problems that are connected with macro systems and that cannot be examined independently of their environment. The importance of the systems view is that it can usually increase insight and understanding for the decision maker in need of a total view of his organization and allows the administrator to:

- evaluate existing conditions,

- change and improve the current state of the process,

- design and add something new to the process to stimulate performance to a more optimum level.

The five major characteristics of the systems approach are that it is organized, creative, empirical, theoretical, and pragmatic.

No matter what the problem is or what the desired form of the solution, the systems approach may be identified as containing the same four basic steps: problem formulation, modeling, analysis and optimization, and implementation.

1. *Problem formulation* is the first and most difficult step, usually requiring about three quarters of the total effort expended in the analysis. It requires a deep understanding of the total problem in the form of verbal descriptions that permit quantification of the significant features. If we wanted to study

the outcome of the delivery of health service to a particular segment of the population, we would have to perform these tasks:
  a. identify all involved decision makers
  b. determine the decision makers' range of alternative actions
  c. determine the consequences of each action in terms of the goals and value structure of the decision maker
  d. include the influence of the total environment within which the decision process occurs
2. *Modeling* refers to the process by which the investigator goes from the real world where the problem has been defined to the abstract world of the model where the analysis will be accomplished. The model is a representation of reality and can be manipulated in ways the actual entities and situations cannot. Model formation is based on maintaining a sensitive balance between inclusion of only the essential reality aspects in the model and limitation of model complexity by the practical considerations of existing theoretical tools, computation time, and data availability.
3. In *analysis and optimization* the model is analyzed with a suitable set of tools in order to find the best strategy for resolving the research problem within the domain of the model. The most common options are analytical techniques or a computer simulation.
4. The final step, *implementation,* is the procedure by which the results determined from the model are translated as a set of actions and transported to the real world.

These four steps of the systems approach, in effect, answer the following five questions in a way that is more specific about the tasks to be accomplished.

1. What is the state of things? Here we are required to select entities of the system, list their attributes, identify activities that can cause changes, and then gather data that provides the attributes' values and defines the relationship involved in the activities. No evaluation is involved.
2. What is the status of things? To answer this question we must utilize an evaluation methodology, and system performance must be measured against some visible, generally accepted standard.
3. What is wrong (or right) with the system? We will answer this question by doing some form of analysis to isolate the difficulties or, if the evaluation was positive, to isolate the critical factors contributing to the success.
4. What can we do about it? To resolve any troubles in the system, we must make a series of recommendations cast in a useful form for the person or agency that has the power to act upon them.
5. How can we promote or advocate our results? The answer to this last question suggests that the investigator should be willing to take responsibil-

ity for injecting himself into the policy making process. The implication for scientists is that they leave their traditional role of neutrality. The intention of this step is that the collaboration of resource people doing the work will make a commitment for positive utilization of their results.

The invocation of the systems approach assures that one or more of the following advantages will be realized (Lapatra, 1975, pp. 10-12).

- Insight and understanding will be achieved for the process being studied.

- Predictions for future states of the system can be made.

- The principles for the designated organizations possessing certain properties and modes of operation can be established.

- Modeling provides a special contribution to the techniques of measurements in social processes.

A final advantage may also be stated in that the health care manager employing this approach is supporting the objectives of effectiveness and efficiency, so essential in the management of any system or resource such as time.

The elements of a systematic problem-solving process for health care administrators consist of four essential steps (Bennett, 1978, p. 197):

1. Recognition. This includes identification, selection, and definition of the existing problem situation.
2. Examination. This refers to the collection and analysis of all relevant facts of the present situation and the development of possible alternative solutions.
3. Evaluation. This includes an evaluation of the various alternatives under consideration and the reaching of a decision as to the best and most effective method available.
4. Installation. This involves the planning, installation, and maintenance of the new and improved method.

Wren (1974, pp. 64-65) also introduced a ten-step systems decision-making process for hospital administrators similar to Bennett's problem-solving paradigm:

1. Become aware of the problem.
2. Investigate the nature of the problem.
3. Determine the objective of the solution desired in light of total organizational objectives.
4. Determine alternative solutions.

5. Weigh the consequences and the relative efficiency of each alternative solution.
6. Try out various alternatives.
7. Select the best alternative solution.
8. Implement the decision.
9. Check up on the solution.
10. Finally, change, correct, or even withdraw the solution if evaluation shows that it is not working or was not the best answer.

The classification of systems is important for the health care administrator who must evaluate social processes, because the resulting system arrangements indicate which quantitative tools the models may use:

1. *Linear or Nonlinear*—This is when the operation can be characterized by linear differential equations. Most processes are nonlinear, and linear approximations are frequently used to deal with them. A physical way to think of the nonlinear is the effect achieved when a component in the system changes its characteristics because of the magnitude of the inputs applied to it. For example, most physicians carrying a very heavy patient load will function differently in several personal dimensions when they have half as many patients. The mathematics associated with analyzing nonlinear systems is very difficult.
2. *Continuous or Discrete*—This depends on whether the operation in time is continuous or intermittent. A student health clinic which is open only at specific, limited times operates discretely, while an emergency service open 24 hours a day is continuous.
3. *Constant or Time Varying*—A system is described as being constant if the system parameters are unchanging with time. Peoples' attitudes change frequently and sometimes cyclically because of the alteration of multiple external conditions. Physical structures such as long distance telephone circuits change from day to night operations as a consequence of temperature changes. If the system parameters are time varying, the mathematics is more difficult.
4. *Lumped or Distributed*—This refers to the spatial distribution of the process represented by the system. A person receiving a rather detailed physical examination must frequently travel to several offices and laboratories in order to complete it, while a multiphasic examination concentrated at one location represents a lumped counterpart to the distributed first case.
5. *Probabilistic or Deterministic*—If there are any uncertainties regarding the magnitude of a variable quantity at a specific point in time, the system is probabilistic or nondeterministic. The number of patients per month who appear with a specific illness cannot be known with certainty, and so

statistical techniques must be used. If an outpatient clinic maintains a rigid schedule with only so many time slots available, then the monthly patient load can be known with certainty (Lapatra, 1975, p. 16).

In addition to the quantitative systems approach, the health care administrator has other processes and techniques that are intended to help clarify priorities and save time via systems theory. Business gaming is one of the techniques used in the decision-making process.

## GAMING

This decision-making technique is a systematic method to deal with complexity. It permits reality-oriented interaction to occur within a simulated organizational environment in which controls can be exercised by the participants. The settings are unstructured and the process of planning is encouraged for the participants. This simulation also saves time usually lost by poor planning during the initial investment in the technique.

The steps required to construct a game are similar to the basic steps of the systems approach.

1. There must be significant understanding of the phenomenon being investigated.
2. With the information of step 1, a model must be constructed that can be controlled, manipulated, and analyzed.
3. The model of step 2 must be stored in a digital computer.
4. Suitable experiments for the game must be designed and the output arranged so that the game results can be appropriately displayed.

Horvath has suggested that, because of the difficulty of modeling the delivery of health services, a set of rules for a game is a way of simulating the identifiable major interactions (Horvath, 1966). The minimum payoff from this approach would be the acquisition of practical insight and the opportunity to refine a speculative primitive model.

The rules of a health system game can be formulated based on the cooperation of public health officials, administrators, health system research workers, practitioners, and representatives of the consuming public. Under a wide variety of stimuli, an agreed-upon code of behavior of the different components of the system can be obtained. This can be done by collecting statistical data, conducting experiments, and utilizing the estimates of a representative group of experts (Lapatra, 1975, p. 20).

## (PPBS) PLANNING, PROGRAMMING, AND BUDGETING SYSTEM

This technique can ascertain the most efficient resource allocation in order to achieve goals that can be quantified.

An alternative to measuring benefits is to measure *effects*. In cost-effectiveness analysis the intent is to determine the least costly method of achieving a desired effect for some fixed amount of resources. The assumptions necessary to use cost-effectiveness analysis are:

- The effects must be measurable.

- The input necessary to produce the desired effects must be measurable.

- A discount mechanism must be available in order to compare present and future costs.

A way of examining health status is to consider the patient flowing through broadly defined stages according to the judgment of the professional treating the patient. This is quite similar to a production process. One version of this approach is to measure patient flow in nine functional areas: medical, dental, nursing, nutritional, social service, psychological, speech and hearing, physical therapy, and occupational therapy. As the patient goes through each area, the following steps are accomplished (Lapatra, 1975, p. 22):

- registration

- health assessment

- treatment

- health supervision.

An important aspect of the flow approach which we may call a model is that the outputs are not laboratory tests, physician hours, filled prescriptions, or nurses' salaries. These are all inputs. Rather, people and their health status are the outputs of the model. Thus, conventional dimensions by themselves are not adequate to utilize cost-effectiveness analysis. A quarterly report lists the flow of patients through each stage and the related supportive flow of resources. All the inputs can be given in terms of dollars; therefore, the average cost per patient per process stage may be computed. For different health service settings, comparisons can be made of resource use, disease distributions, and the effect on cost variation. If sufficient data is available for the flow model so that the input and output number of patients is known for all stages, then, depending on the characteristics of the flow, predictions can be possible. For example, if it turned out that changes in patient flow were cyclical in nature and the cycles could be characterized so that predictions could be made, then this information would be the basis for an analysis of alternative uses of input resources (Lapatra, 1975, p. 23). The flow approach yields these indicators needed for the planning and ultimate controlling of health care: cost per patient, cost per disease, income per disease, cost per state, and output measures of patient flow. This also leads to an efficient management approach and time-effective process.

A key to this planning system is feedback. Cybernetics, the study of methods of feedback control, is an important part of systems review and evaluation. A corrective device is needed to get the system back on course, and the control mechanism working at the point of output provides the control information the manager needs to do this. As the manager examines and evaluates results of his work unit against established levels of expectation, he obtains the kinds of information that show him how well or how poorly his systems area is performing, in terms of these expected achievements. This flow of information is then fed back into the system to determine whether or not input policies and practices need correcting, whether or not purposes require modification, and whether or not the systems activity or use of resources needs further examination and improvement.

This concept of control and correction is applicable to all three levels of concern embraced by systems purposes. As the manager considers the work unit's purposes, he will need to make continual use of the feedback channels of information. As he periodically examines and evaluates progress in achieving the work unit's objectives, the manager will find feedback control helpful in making sure he considers all elements of the system as they affect levels of objective achievement. Finally, as he engages in specific improvement projects, he will again need to use feedback as he documents the problem definition and evaluates the effectiveness of improvement (Bennett, 1978, p. 147).

## STRATEGIC PLANNING

No discussion of planning as a decision-making process and effective managerial tool can be complete without examining strategic planning.

Planning activities can be divided into two types: tactical planning and strategic planning. Strategic planning is long-range planning that focuses on the organization as a whole. Long-range usually is defined as a period of time extending about three to five years into the future; therefore, managers are trying to determine what their organization should do to be successful at some point three to five years in the future.

Successful strategic planning must focus on such factors as (1) organizational environment, (2) the difference between where the organization is and where it wants to go, (3) organizational purpose, (4) organizational goals, and (5) strengths and weaknesses of the organization as it presently exists. How far into the future should managers extend their strategic planning? The commitment principle suggests managers should commit resources for planning only if they can antici- pate, in the foreseeable future, a return on planning expenses as a result of the long-range planning analysis. Realistically, planning costs are an investment and, therefore, should not be incurred unless a reasonable return on that investment is anticipated.

Tactical planning is short-range planning that emphasizes current operations of various parts of the organization. Short-range is defined as a period of time extending only about one year or less into the future. Strategic and tactical planning complement each other. They can be examined independently but can't be responsible for strategic plans, while middle managers carry out tactical plans.

Drucker describes strategic planning as the continuous process of making present entrepreneurial (risk-taking) decisions systematically and with the greatest knowledge of their futurity; organizing systematically the efforts needed to carry out these decisions; and measuring the results of these decisions against the expectations through organized, systematic feedback (Drucker, 1974, p. 125).

Glueck and Mankin (1975) describe strategic planning and its importance: Strategic planning is that set of decisions and actions which leads to the develop- ment of an effective strategy. The best way to describe strategic planning in more detail is to analyze the key words and phrases contained within this definition.

A strategy is a unified, comprehensive, and integrated plan designed to assure that the basic objectives of the enterprise are achieved. The objectives are the basic economic and social purposes for which the enterprise exists. For a hospital, examples of objectives are quality patient care, excess revenues over costs, and provision of low cost health care.

Strategy is the *means* used to achieve the ends (objectives). A strategy is not just any plan, however. A strategy is comprehensive: It covers all major aspects of the hospital. A strategy is integrated: All the parts of the plan are compatible with each other and fit together well.

Strategic planning is a continuous process, adapting to changing circumstances. The output of strategic planning is not a document or plan: It is a managerial philosophy. Because strategic planning is a philosophy and not a research report, top management is primarily involved with the decision process, leaving the details and the implementation for middle management (Glueck & Mankin, 1975, p. 408).

However, hospitals are not like other businesses since they operate with a triad of top managers consisting of administrators, trustees, and medical staff. These are three diverse power sources, and management by cooperation (Appelbaum, 1977, p. 19) is a prime objective in the quest for effectiveness.

Planning starts with the objectives of the business. In each area of objectives, the question needs to be asked: "What do we have to do now to attain our objectives tomorrow?" The first thing to do to attain tomorrow is always to be sloughing off yesterday. Most plans concern themselves only with the new and additional things that have to be done—new products, new processes, new markets, and so on. But the key to doing something different tomorrow is getting rid of the no longer productive, the obsolescent, the obsolete.

The first step in planning is to ask of any activity, and product, any process or market: "If we were not committed to this today, would we go into it?" If the answer is no, one says, "How can we get out—fast?"

Systematic sloughing off of yesterday is a plan by itself—and adequate in many businesses. It will force thinking and action. It will make available personnel and money for new things. It will create willingness to act.

Conversely, the plan that provides only for doing additional and new things without provision for sloughing off old and tired ones is unlikely to have results. It will remain a plan and never become reality. Getting rid of yesterday is the decision that most long-range plans in business (and even more in government) never tackle—which may be the main reason for their futility (Drucker, 1974, p. 126).

The foundation for planning is to make current decisions with an understanding of their future. The view of the future determines the span of time with which administrators are always grappling. Results requiring long incubation periods can be achieved only if they are conceptualized and acted upon quite early in the process. Long-range planning actually connotes some view of the future, since managers are always juggling current activities with targets to be achieved in a future time period. But planning is only effective if it becomes work that can be measured at a later date for completion and achievement. The true test of a plan is the commitment of resources (human and financial) to action that is intended to accrue results in the future. Commitment usually results in achievable plans.

It is important to note that strategic planning is not a substitution of facts for good judgment or a substitution of management science for management art. This process actually increases the importance of the manager's role since the systematic organization of the function of planning and supply of data strengthens the decision-making prowess of the manager. Successful strategic planning in hospitals is usually accomplished by the chief administrator, who always needs the cooperation of the board and medical staff. Therefore, cooperation and not quantifiable results is the barometer for success within this dynamic, complex environment.

In projecting future demands, Glueck and Mankin (1975, pp. 409-410) questioned health care administrators with regard to their strategic planning and projections regarding future contingencies affecting their operation and time commitments:

When the administrators were asked what the trend of the health care industry seemed to be over the last 10 years, two-thirds said that more government involvement (socialized medicine) was in prospect. One-third felt that there was increasing pressure from clients. Government intervention was considered something that the administrators could adapt to, but the consumerist movement was of concern to the administrators in that there were no evident strategic changes or choices which they felt would meet this challenge.

The majority of hospital administrators felt that National Health Insurance and Professional Standards Review Organizations were going to have the greatest future effect on their institution. . . . Ninety-three percent of the administrators held regularly scheduled meetings to discuss future strategies or major strategic choices. Only one adminstrator said he held daily meetings while one-third of the administrators (53%) held monthly meetings. These meetings were usually titled department head meetings in which problems and proposals were brought forth for discussion. The weekly meetings were most often administrative meetings in which only a few of the top department heads were present along with the administrator and his staff.

The strategic planning model and approach is conducive to effective management, efficient operation, and conservation of resources (time and manpower commitments). This technique and philosophy is comprehensive, and a desirable component of the integral health care system.

---

## REFERENCES

Appelbaum, S.H. Management by cooperation: The views of seven chief executive officers. *University of Michigan Business Review,* November 1977, *24*(6), 19.

Archibald, R.D., & Villoria, R.L. *Network based management systems (PERT-CPM).* New York: John Wiley and Sons, 1967.

Bennett, A.C. *Improving management performance in health care institutions: A total systems approach.* Chicago: American Hospital Association, 1978.

Dittrich, J.E., Lang, J.R., & White, S.E. Nurses' management problems and their training implications. *Personnel Journal,* May 1979, *58*(5), 314.

Drucker, P.F. *Management: Tasks, responsibilities, practices.* New York: Harper and Row, 1974.

Gantt, H.L. *Organizing for work.* New York: Harcourt & Brace, 1919.

Glueck, W.F., & Mankin, D.C. Strategic planning in the hospital setting. *Proceedings of the 35th Annual Meeting of the Academy of Management,* 1975, 408-410.

Horvath, W.J. The systems approach to the national health problem. *Management Science,* October 1966, *12*(10).

Lapatra, J.W. *Health care delivery systems*. Springfield, Ill.: Charles C. Thomas, 1975.

Parkinson, C.N. *Parkinson's law*. Boston: Houghton Mifflin Co., 1957.

Parkinson, C.N. *The law of delay*. Boston: Houghton Mifflin Co., 1971.

Wren, D.A. *The evolution of management thought*. New York: Ronald Press, 1972.

Wren, G.R. *Modern health administration*. Athens: University of Georgia Press, 1974.

# Chapter 5

# Managing Productivity

## TIME MANAGEMENT HIGHLIGHTS

1. Productivity is the ratio between the output and the factors that have contributed to the input usually expressed as:

$$\text{Productivity} = \frac{\text{output}}{\text{input}}$$

2. The complexity of the hospital operation makes it difficult to isolate time as a separate input. Nevertheless, certain methods for measuring hospital productivity have bearing on the output effect.

3. Organizational efficiency refers to the way in which the resources of an organization are arranged. The three components of this measure are coordination, controls, and goals to achieve the desired health status of the community. Quality of health in an area can be derived from indexes of unnecessary disease, disability, and untimely death.

4. Worker productivity is often the result of management productivity. Most problems of productivity have their source in managerial decisions concerning job definitions, controls, and work flow.

5. A quality-productivity program frees top management for long-range planning and still permits the close monitoring of day-to-day operations by integrating the activities between health care departments.

6. A myth exists that increased productivity reduces the quality of health care. Not only is this not true, but research indicates that increased quality can be consistent with increased productivity; increases in total hospital productivity result in decreased costs.

7. Physician productivity is important since the greatest amount of time is required of physicians between the ages of 30 to 40 when their stress and mortality rates are at a peak.

8. What is important in the productivity of physicians is not the size of their firms as measured by the quantity of physicians employed, but the use of larger numbers of auxiliary personnel and the management principle of task delegation.
9. Value analysis is another technique to be considered since it is a method of securing the same or better performance of a function or activity at a lesser total cost. It demands an objective ongoing evaluation and review of innovative ideas, alternative procedures, and other changes which may produce positive results for all involved. It provides more effective time management by identifying costly usage of time while recommending new, viable, more productive alternatives.

The management of time is a crucial task and activity for the health care administrator who is charged with maximizing productivity, maintaining high quality patient care, and planning for institutional perpetuation. Since time is one of the essential resources, it must be managed similarly to the factors of production. Productivity has a close linkage to time since both factors are usually evaluated along similar continuums. However, the measurement of managerial productivity is a complex task. Collectively, management performance in an organization can be appraised by comparing it to that of similar organizations. Such indexes as return on equity, revenue per customer, expenditure per employee, and profit per invested dollar are relevant here. This is somewhat difficult to do in a health care setting, but not impossible.

On an individual basis, however, managers must be appraised by comparing their performance to a standard. In order to do this effectively, reasonable performance objectives must be operationally defined and performance results must be clearly measured against the original objectives. Studies of managerial leadership styles have shown that effective leadership, as measured by worker attitudes and increased productivity, is a function of the interaction between the manager and his subordinates. There is no simple formula to describe the interaction. The complex health care climate further complicates this analysis.

Predicting managerial success and productivity also requires an objective analysis of desirable performance outcomes and the behaviors necessary to achieve these outcomes. Assessment centers have attempted to do this by simulating tasks that are similar to the real task involved in adequate job performance. While the evidence is not conclusive, these procedures do appear to be useful. However, this approach will not be examined in this book.

A number of approaches have been developed to increase managerial productivity. Management development programs, for example, have been designed to produce more effective managers. Their success, however, often depends on how clearly their goals are defined and on how accurately their outcomes are measured. Some have focused upon time management.

Management by Objectives (MBO) programs specifically deal with the objective delineation of desirable goals and the methods needed to achieve them. The principles of behavior theory dictate that rewards must be contingent upon objectively defined and measured behaviors. Data indicate that the combination of a good MBO program and contingent reinforcement may be a powerful tool in the effort to improve managerial performance, productivity, and time utilization. One of the ways to examine the effective utilization of time is to explore the dimensions of productivity that are an integral part of the health care administrator's task, responsibility, and domain. These dimensions include output, input, efficiency, quality, and the management process.

## PRODUCTIVITY

The American Hospital Association (1973) states, "Productivity is the ratio between the goods or services produced (output) and the factors that have contributed to the production (input). It is usually expressed in terms of output per so many dollars of capital invested, per so many pounds of raw material, or per so many manhours, provided the quality of output can be considered uniform." In this definition two very important aspects have been properly recognized. The first is that depending upon what is being measured, the units of the ratio may appropriately vary. For example, the cost of a piece of automated laboratory equipment is a valid input (which can, in fact, be equated with the value of the labor it replaces). The second aspect is that the quality of the output has been introduced as a parameter, i.e., a quantity that may be assigned a desired value. Productivity includes measurement variables and standards:

- *Measurement Variables:* Activities on which judgment or decision can be based. Both qualitative and quantitative measurement variables can be used, but quantitative variables are less subjective. Examples of measurement variables are sterility of instrument trays, accuracy of accounting records, cleanliness of patient rooms, and preparation minutes per tray pack.

- *Standards:* Specific values of measurement variables. Each quality and productivity measurement variable can have specific levels or standards established as acceptable and unacceptable. Examples of standards are 95 percent acceptably cleaned rooms or five instrument trays packed per hour.

Productivity is actually a measure of the relationship between output and input when both are expressed in real physical value terms:

$$\text{Productivity} = \frac{\text{total output}}{\text{total input}}$$

When only one output relates uniquely to only one input so that there is a one-to-one correspondence between them, the conceptual and operational problems of measurement are considerably simplified. But severe problems may arise when the outputs, the inputs, or both, are multiple. It is important to examine both output and input dimensions of productivity in order to understand the resultants of efficiency-effectiveness which become illuminated when time management within the health care institution is demanded.

## What Is Output?

The first issue in the measurement of productivity is the specification of the product. Generally, where the product is concrete, this is not a matter of great difficulty. In medical care, on the other hand, the nature of the product remains a matter for debate and disagreement. In examining the problem, one encounters once again the curious duality of process and outcome to which we shall have occasion to return repeatedly. Those who are oriented to process define the product of the medical care system as medical care. They are concerned, therefore, with identifying the specific contribution of the service-producing units (for example, the physician) to the medical care process. Those who are oriented to outcome are inclined to consider the process of medical care as an intermediate input, and to emphasize the end results of care expressed as some state of health or well-being in the client (Donabedian, 1973, p. 250).

Another aspect of the definition of output pertains to the manner in which standby capacity is to be handled. Whenever services provided or cases processed are used as the measure of output, no account is taken of the investment in holding hospital beds or ambulatory care personnel and facilities ready for action when the call for their services arises. As we shall see, this is a question that has attracted considerable attention where hospitals are concerned. This is because of the preponderant magnitude of fixed costs, as compared to variable costs, in hospital operations. The same kinds of considerations should, however, also be applicable to evaluating the productivity of other resources, including that of physicians in office practice. For example, a research study reported that in one group practice each physician put in 42 hours of work plus 28 hours of "active standby on call" per week (Wolfe, et al., 1968, p. 119). This means that 40 percent of the physician's weekly output is in standby services. Yet the usual measures of physician output (and most measures of hospital output) ignore the standby service component. One important reason may be the difficulty of estimating what amount of standby service is necessary and legitimate, and what amount merely represents oversupply (Donabedian, p. 252).

## What Is Input?

Both outputs and inputs are as similar and as different as two sides of a coin. However, an input that requires special attention is *time*. Physicians may increase their production either by working longer hours or by organizing their work in a way that permits them to accomplish more during a given period of time. Accordingly, Garbarino (1960, p. 47) has distinguished the "output effect," which is the effect of operating at different percentages of capacity, and the "methods effect," which is the effect of changing methods of production.

It is standard to express the productivity of labor in terms of a fixed unit, usually a manhour. This excludes the effect of longer or shorter hours of work except as they indirectly influence performance while at work. In analogous studies of the productivity of health manpower, it would be useful to distinguish the two factors of "output" and "method" and to gauge their separate effects on production. This is especially important because hours of work are more subject to variation in independent practice. In all instances it should be made clear whether the measure of health manpower productivity that is used includes or excludes variation in time as an input. In studies of the productivity of hospitals, the time factor is usually not recognized as a separable input. This may be because the hospital is supposed to operate at peak capacity round the clock, every day of the week—an assumption that is known not to be true. Furthermore, the complexity of the hospital operation would make it difficult to isolate time as a separate input. Nevertheless, certain variations in the methods for measuring hospital productivity have a bearing on the "output effect" (Donabedian, 1973, p. 256). It appears to be a fact that the individual contribution of private practice physicians often determines the productivity of the hospital. Also, the productivity of private practice physicians is directly influenced by the way in which they utilize the hospital. The narrow preoccupation with the productivity of the physician alone or of the hospital alone will not provide incentives for maximizing the joint productivity of both (Johnson, 1969, p. 59). A basic input/output system model is shown in Figure 5-1 to offer an overview of the total system and its elements.

In any work situation, the common denominator is an input, one or more steps of processing, and an output. The activities of each functional area all have purposes that utilize various resources for their fulfillment. When the three elements of work occur—namely, when work is accepted (input), processed (system activity), and finished (output) by a department—there exists a work-producing unit, which may be the patient seen, the test completed, the report sent out, the film exposed, and so forth (Bennett, 1978, p. 140). Examples of work-producing units are included in Table 5-1.

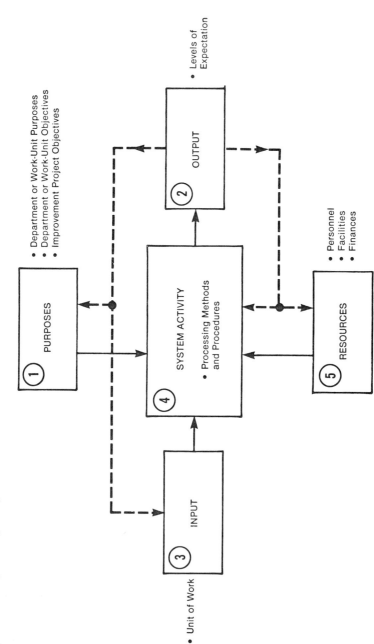

**Figure 5-1** Input/Output System Model

*Source:* A.E. Bennett, *Improving Management Performance in Health Care Institutions*, 1978, p. 114. Used by permission of American Hospital Association.

**Table 5-1**  Work-Producing Units

| Department or Unit | Input | Process | Output |
|---|---|---|---|
| Radiology department | Patient test requisition | Position patient<br>Expose plate<br>Develop plate<br>Interpret plate | Test report |
| Microbiology laboratory | Specimen test requisition | Plate for culture<br>Incubate<br>Examine plate<br>Record findings | Test report |
| Admitting | Individual requiring medical treatment | Interview individual<br>Initiate needed records and information flow<br>Orient patient<br>Transport patient | Fully admitted patient |
| ECG | Patient test requisition | Apply electrodes<br>Run test<br>Examine strip | Test report |
| Central sterile supply | Used needles | Clean<br>Sharpen<br>Pack<br>Sterilize | Packaged sterile needles |

The primary purpose of the basic model shown in Table 5-1 is to provide managers at all levels an integrated means by which the purposes, goals, or objectives of the hospital, or any functional unit of it, can be met according to rules (or policies and decisions); this involves using several types of input (or things to be dealt with) to produce a series of processing steps, with one or more types of output (results accomplished or information made available), all within the constraints of available resources (things, people, money, materials, space, skills, or information) (Bennett, p. 142).

## What Is Efficiency?

In its simplest form, organizational efficiency refers to the way in which the resources of an organization are arranged. In the maximally efficient organization the resources (whether land, labor, capital, goodwill, or any combination thereof) are so arranged that no other method would produce as profitable a return. (Return can refer to profitability, quality of health care, election of a political candidate, or whatever the goal of a given organization.)

In order to operationalize this concept, it is necessary to define organizational goals, measure the degree of goal attainment as well as the value of organizational resources, and know all possible alternative arrangements for these resources. Short of such perfection, researchers have measured "efficiency" and labeled their findings variously as efficiency, quality, performance, effectiveness, goal achievement, or success.

Efficiency is generally measured by the ratio of outputs (returns, benefits) to inputs (costs, effort). Ideally all inputs and outputs are included (Becker & Neuhauser, 1975, p. 40). There appear to be three components to organizational efficiency. These are "coordination" and "control" over the resources needed to achieve some "goal."

In looking at problems of control and coordination, some theorists will concentrate on organizational structure, such as the problems of communication, distribution of power, and centralization. Others will look at technology, such as the substitution of capital for labor or man-machine relationships. Still others will look at the human factors, such as managerial style, morale, motivation, and role definition. We must deal with structure and managerial style and view them as the same variable—e.g., degree to which specified procedures determine not only authority patterns but structural patterns as well (Becker & Neuhauser, p. 168).

## What Is Quality?

The ultimate measure of quality of the health care system is the health status of the community. Quality of health in an area can be derived from indexes of unnecessary disease, unnecessary disability, and unnecessary untimely death (Rutstein, 1974). However, such measures of quality have undefined relationships with the services provided by specific hospital departments. Hence, measures should be used that are more specific to the services being provided by the respective physicians or departments.

A definition of quality related to production is: "The quality of a product or service is expressed in terms of a given set of attributes that are required to meet the . . . needs for which the product or service is created" (Gavett, 1968).

Quality control systems exist and can be developed both for medical care provided by physicians and for services provided by hospital departments. Some departments, such as nuclear medicine and tissue pathology, have strong medical components.

## What Is Hospital Output?

The hospital has many products, only one of which is patient care. Patient care itself is divisible into many components. The argument that various components of office care should be kept separate and treated as products, each of which has a separate production function, should apply with even greater force to the hospital. This is because hospital care has an even larger number of separable patient care components and is formally organized into fairly autonomous units or departments. The hospital is actually a multiproduct (multiservice) health plant. Each of its independent units—for example, laboratory, radiology, dietary—produces an independent microproduct. There are other axes of classification—for example, medical service, nursing service, housekeeping service, and administration. The patient care units are themselves organized into departments such as medicine, surgery, pediatrics, obstetrics-gynecology, and newborn nursery. It is not only possible, but very likely, that productivities in these various subunits have experienced different trends and are currently different from each other, within a given hospital as well as among hospitals. Such differences arise from a variety of factors, which include degrees of administrative rationalization, manpower differentiation, and substitution (as in nursing), and mechanization or automation (as in laboratory services) (Donabedian, 1973, p. 264).

It is clear that the measurement variables and standards of productivity, along with output, input, efficiency, and quality are components of the total management process which is our concern in the management of time for the health care professional.

## THE MANAGEMENT PROCESS—KEY LINK IN PRODUCTIVITY

Several research studies have examined productivity and organization management. The findings are most interesting to consider in the quest for effectiveness and efficiency.

It was found in one study (Sayles, 1973, pp. 57-58) that productivity, like profitability, is the result of a large number of decisions and organizational elements. Worker productivity is often the result of management productivity. Most problems of productivity have their source in managerial decisions concerning job definitions, controls, and work flow. The manager must design jobs so that the work flows regularly and continuously. Regularity, not speed, is the source of high productivity. There is a direct link in this recommendation between productivity and the efficient management of resources (time).

In another study (Dobbs, 1976), the researchers found that quite often, in the push for productivity, managers overlook the really essential element: people. Productivity measures what is produced in relation to what is consumed in order to produce it. Most programs aimed at increasing productivity are useless without employee cooperation. Many people will resist changes of any kind because they fear job loss, a speedup, relocation, or the unknown. Employees want to know what's in it for them.

People costs, as a key factor in calculating productivity, are comprised of more than salaries and benefits (costs of absenteeism, turnover costs, decreased morale and loyalty, and so forth).

It was recommended that the following steps be followed by managers trying to increase productivity:

1. Make a diagnosis of on-the-job problems (candid interview).
2. Invest in sound, well-thought-out formal training.
3. Involve subordinates.
4. Make use of performance appraisals and objectives.
5. Don't overlook training for subordinate supervisors or yourself.

Lack of employee cooperation often leads to dysfunctional and counterproductive conflict for management which is difficult to resolve. Even the resolution is costly from a time perspective.

An evaluation of management is essentially an appraisal of past performance and future probable performance in the context of the industry environment. The appraisal would include a consideration of long-term and recent rates of return on equity and market penetration in relation to competitors or the industry as a whole. Trends, averages, and variances of these elements should be considered. In special cases, the relative profit margin performance might also be relevant. Qualitative impressions are also an integral part of the process, and these might include a review of successor management programs, product and marketing strategies, and indications of management's general imagination and aggressiveness as contrasted to possible complacency and inertia (Hayes, 1968, pp. 39-42). The evaluation process includes measures of efficiency as well as effectiveness. The dimension of time as a scarce resource is also an index to determine the performance and productivity of management.

It is also essential to examine the impact of managerial style upon productivity since it is the manager of the institution who establishes the model for efficient management. Researchers (Misumi & Shirakashi, 1966) experimentally set up three types of supervision: goal-achievement oriented (type P), process-maintenance oriented (type M), and a combination of the two (type PM). Under these varying supervisory conditions, three subjects performed the simple task of counting holes punched in IBM cards. Group productivity was the total number of cards in which the holes had been counted accurately in 50 minutes.

Results indicated that the P, M, and PM styles of the first-line supervisors were verified by the perceptions of the subjects and by observers' records. Productivity was highest under first-line supervisors of PM type, second under P type, and lowest under M type. Degree of interest in the task was significantly higher under the PM type than under the P or M types. Attitudes towards the supervisors were significantly more favorable under PM than under P.

The authors conclude that it is when the M function and the P function are combined, thus enabling the former to act as a catalyst on the latter, that they provide optimum stimulation for increments of productivity and morale. It appears that managers who support goal-achievement behavior as a catalyst, develop a structured climate where efficiency and productivity are emphasized.

Another research study (Wofford, 1971) also examined managerial effectiveness. In this study 177 employees from 88 companies in the Dallas-Fort Worth area, ranging in size from 3 to 36,000 employees, served as subjects. The employees rated their work unit's performance in terms of the quantity of its output, the quality of output, and the morale of its members. A composite of the quality and quantity ratings was used as the productivity criterion.

A factor analysis yielded the following factors of managerial behavioral dimensions: group achievement and order, personal enhancement, personal interaction, dynamic achievement, and security and maintenance. These behavioral dimensions accounted for 40 percent of the variance in productivity and 54 percent of the variance in morale. Group achievement and order had the highest corrected correlation with the productivity criterion, and security and maintenance and personal interaction had the highest corrected correlation with morale. Personal enhancement had a strong negative relationship to both criteria.

Eighteen situational variables were selected for measurement and subjected to a factor analysis, yielding the following five factors: centralization and work evaluation (decision-making power and closeness of supervisory control), organizational complexity, size and structure, group structure of the work unit, and organizational layering and communication.

This study presented the complex relationships between the dimension of managerial behavior and its relationship to productivity and morale when moderated by the above situational factors. The managerial behavioral dimensions most effective for productivity, however, are not the most effective for morale.

These studies do illuminate the linkage between efficiency, productivity, and the management process. This process is crucial to understanding the balancing of productivity and quality in a health care institution.

The complete management process (or system) contains four types of activities: research and development, planning, operations, and review (Malcolm & Rowe, 1960). Research and development investigates innovations and solutions to problems. Planning incorporates research and development innovations and solutions, plus review actions, into the future operations. Operations use input resources and plans to produce desired results or outputs. *Review assesses the degree to which outputs meet the established objectives or standards.* This review leads to recommended actions for both planning and operations.

The typical management of a hospital department focuses on the operation of the department, with informal monitoring and complaints serving as the quality control process. This is simple but has many disadvantages.

However, the management of a hospital department using an existing productivity and/or quality system is a significant improvement with the following advantages:

1. Standards of productivity and/or quality are used to judge departmental performance.
2. Review is done consistently for quality and/or productivity for the departments on the system.
3. Actions based on review serve as inputs to both planning and operations.
4. Data reported by the monitoring system allow hospital administration to monitor productivity and/or quality.
5. Planning can be done using estimated workloads and the standards of production. In most cases, the planning is limited to budget planning.
6. Systems are relatively easy to implement and allow for the control of many "time" elements and components. However, some existing systems still have obvious shortcomings.

## THE QUALITY-PRODUCTIVITY MANAGEMENT PROGRAM

To further improve the cost-effectiveness of a community hospital's provision of high quality medical care, and to maintain the level of improvement already accomplished, the administration may require a more sophisticated ongoing administrative tool to transfer the day-to-day management of departments and systems to the middle managers. This tool would free top management time for long-range planning and still allow top managers to closely monitor day-to-day operations. To provide such a tool, the administration may develop and implement a major new quality-productivity program.

Such a quality-productivity program might consist of two major innovations:

1. Integration of quality and productivity measurement of hospital departments.
2. Inclusion of inter-department interaction in the quality and productivity measurement system.

There are several community-level concerns that support and indicate the need for the development of such a program. Hospital costs continue to increase. It is clear that new approaches must be developed to contain these costs, yet cost containment must not be effected at the expense of quality of care. It is necessary, however, to consider whether the quality of care provided is in fact too high and thus too costly. The determination of this aspect of the problem must come through a quality measurement system such as the community hospital model. This program links quality measurement with productivity measurement so that a more appropriate balance can be established and maintained between the quality of care provided and the cost of that care.

The impact of a carefully developed and implemented quality-productivity program will be significant. Most importantly, to patients, quality of service will be monitored so that it can be maintained at consistently high levels while productivity is increased. The impact on the hospital will be an improved capability for cost-effective operation by use of the system.

Hospital employees and managers will have established standards of performance that have been developed with department head participation. Thus, employees can be treated fairly and consistently. For third party payors, the program will assure a high quality of care for their subscribers, with effective cost control through productivity monitoring.

Figure 5-2 illustrates the management of a hospital department using the community hospital quality-productivity system. The primary advantages of this system are:

1. All departments in the hospital are included in the quality-productivity program.
2. "Network" and hospitalwide systems (such as utilization review, infection control, communications, and information systems) are included in the program.
3. Standards of quality and productivity are used to judge departmental and interdepartmental performance. These standards provide specific achievement goals for departmental and administrative staff.
4. Standards are hospital-specific. Known reasonable standards of quality and productivity are used as a basis for establishing a hospital-specific standard for each of the measurement variables that the hospital chooses to use. The variables involve interactions between departments for which standards have been developed.
5. Review is done consistently for both quality and productivity for all departments and multidepartment systems.
6. Actions based on the review of departments and their interactions serve as inputs to planning and operations of all related departments.
7. Data reported by the monitoring system and interdepartmental task force reports allow hospital administration to monitor quality and productivity and to take appropriate actions to improve both.
8. Planning can be done using estimated workloads and outputs of the quality-productivity monitoring and review. This allows complete planning because all departments and their interactions are included.
9. Review of quality and productivity is integrated.

**Figure 5-2** Management of Hospital Department Using Quality-Productivity System

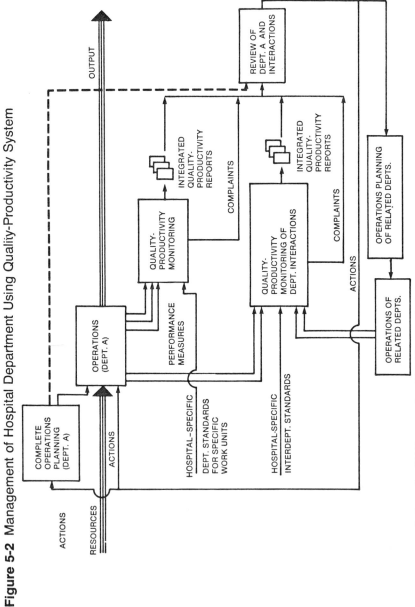

*Source:* Karl G. Bartscht, Chi Systems, Inc. Used by permission.

## Relationship of Quality and Productivity

The relationship of quality and productivity is not easily determined nor consistent. It varies with levels of quality and productivity, and the procedures used by the hospital. A myth exists that increased productivity reduces the quality of care. Not only is this generally *not true,* but the research indicates that *increased quality can be consistent with increased productivity* and increases in total hospital productivity result in decreased cost.

Figure 5-3 illustrates relationships of quality and productivity and their management implications. Starting from current quality and productivity levels, changes in procedures, staffing, and so forth, will cause four types of changes:

1. Quality and productivity up. This is the desired outcome.
2. Quality and productivity down. This is definitely undesirable and should result in a return to at least the previous quality and productivity levels.
3. Quality up and productivity down.
4. Quality down and productivity up.

---

**Figure 5-3** Relationship of Quality and Productivity

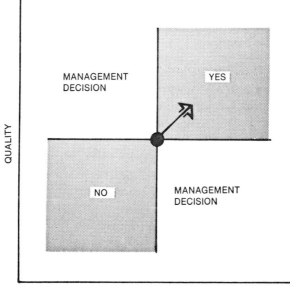

The last two conditions should result in a verification that the observed changes exist and are necessary. Then a management decision must be made concerning the value of the change in quality versus the change in productivity.

Obviously, the difficulty is in knowing where the hospital is currently and monitoring where it will be in the future. This is a major reason for a quality-productivity program that simultaneously measures and integrates quality and productivity. Then as changes in both are planned, the impact on the other can be determined.

## Mini-Case

A specific example can be given to illustrate how to increase both productivity (at decreasing cost) and quality. In many hospitals, physicians write pharmacy orders on the patients' charts. These orders are then transcribed by a ward clerk, checked by the head nurse, and sent to the pharmacy to be filled. Changing the system so that a carbon copy of the physician's order is sent directly to the pharmacy results in the following:

1. decreases in errors in interpreting the physician's order, thus increasing quality
2. reduction of staff time to transcribe and verify the physician's order, which can increase productivity or decrease cost

The steps required to develop a quality-productivity reporting system are presented in Figure 5-4, with the steps required to operate such a system being given in Figure 5-5. The steps required to operate a quality-productivity monitoring system in a typical cost center are presented in Figure 5-6. All serve as models for health care administrators interested in quality-productivity as a component of time management.

**Figure 5-4** Steps to Develop a Quality-Productivity Reporting System

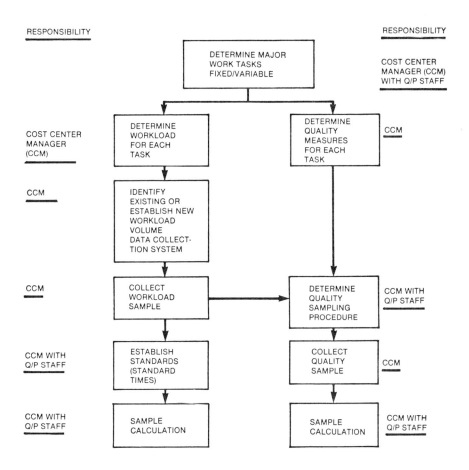

*Source:* Karl G. Bartscht, Chi Systems, Inc. Used by permission.

**Figure 5-5** Steps to Operate a Quality-Productivity Reporting System

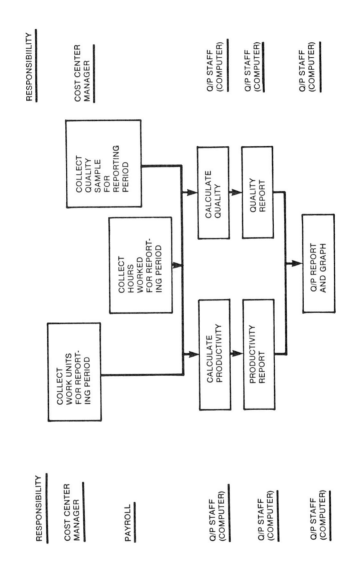

*Source:* Karl G. Bartscht, Chi Systems, Inc. Used by permission.

**Figure 5-6** Steps to Operate a Productivity-Quality Monitoring System in a Typical Cost Center

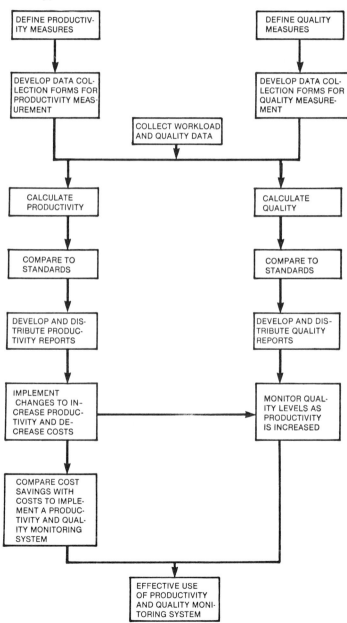

*Source:* Karl G. Bartscht, Chi Systems, Inc. Used by permission.

**Program Uniqueness**

The quality-productivity program is unique in several very important ways, including:

1. *Monitoring both quality and productivity.* The program measures, establishes standards for, and monitors both quality and productivity for all hospital departments. Most existing programs only monitor productivity for a few departments and some monitor quality for a few departments.
2. *Integrating quality and productivity.* The quality measures and productivity measures are integrated for each department. This was difficult but important for consideration of the trade-offs. Integration of quality and productivity is not part of any existing program.
3. *Including network systems.* The quality-productivity program includes interactions that are the specific responsibility of task forces composed of people from the related departments. As an example, consider the situation in which it is desired that an x-ray examination be made of an inpatient. All forms have been properly processed. But before the exam can occur, the patient must be transported from his or her bed to the x-ray department, a function that belongs neither to nursing, the x-ray department, nor the physician. The "network system" here is patient transportation. Other network systems include communications (verbal, print, electronic, recorded); material supply (procurement, reprocessing, storage, distribution); education; and equipment and facility maintenance. No existing system measures quality and productivity of such "network systems," and reflects the performance in departmental reports.
4. *Negotiating hospital-specific standards.* Known reasonable standards for quality and productivity are used as a basis for negotiating a hospital-specific standard for each of the measurement variables used. The reason for hospital-specific standards is that standards are meaningful, acceptable, and useful to department heads and administration.
5. *Educating hospital personnel.* The intention is to improve quality and productivity, not merely buy a statistical reporting system. Seminars, assignments, and private counselling are used to educate department heads and others concerning the goals, measurement process, monitoring system, and methods of improving the current situation.
6. *Prospective budgeting and control.* The quality-productivity program provides an excellent tool for projecting staff needs from expected workload. This can then serve as a basis for an employee incentive program or a hospital prospective reimbursement program.
7. *Planning for hospital.* Planning can be done using estimated workloads, standards, and outputs of the quality-productivity program. This allows

complete planning because all departments and their interactions are included.

8. *Evaluating program.* The impact of the quality-productivity program can be evaluated for one year. This allows time for management changes and the resulting impacts. Evaluation is an important part of any new program and eliminates the wasting of time due to inefficient operations.

## A Case Study—The Housekeeping Department

*Problem*

Housekeeping services at a community hospital had deteriorated to the point where immediate action on the part of the new administration was necessary. Symptoms pointing to poor services and employee dissatisfaction included:

1. Poor general appearance of the entire facility.
2. High frequency of complaints from departments throughout the institution. Complaints referred to inferior cleaning and poor attitude on the part of housekeeping employees.
3. High turnover of personnel.
4. Low morale on the part of housekeeping personnel.
5. Poor appearance of cleaning equipment.

An investigation of the department and a hospitalwide opinion survey of housekeeping services produced the following results:

1. Housekeeping was providing cleaning services on a poor to fair basis. In a hospital this is totally unacceptable.
2. The quality control program being utilized was totally ineffective and improperly structured as evidenced by the following:
   a. Supervisors were allowed to perform their own inspections and grade the results.
   b. Inspections were performed on a selective rather than random basis.
   c. Cleaning frequencies and standards were obtained.
   d. Program output results were deceivingly high.
3. Inservice training was almost nonexistent.
4. Policies and procedures were either outdated or, in many cases, not utilized.
5. Cleaning equipment was to a great extent old and ineffective and poor in appearance.
6. Many of the staff including management and cleaning personnel were not job qualified.
7. Interviews with management and cleaning personnel substantiated low morale and job dissatisfaction.

*Action*

A plan of action was developed immediately thereafter to accomplish the following:

1. Evaluate management and replace as necessary.
2. Evaluate cleaning staff and replace as necessary.
3. Evaluate training programs and update as necessary.
4. Evaluate desired level of cleaning for hospital, review personnel assignments, and update as necessary.
5. Inventory and evaluate cleaning equipment and replace as necessary.
6. Update all cleaning standards and frequencies and redesign the housekeeping quality control program.

The plan of action was put into effect immediately, with the following results produced ten months later.

*Results*

1. *Management Changes:* The program director and two of three supervisors were replaced and the supervisory staff was increased from three to five. One of the key new positions was assistant to the director, whose primary responsibility involves central monitoring of the new quality control program. The other change was assigning a dedicated supervisor responsibility for all project work. The remaining supervisors (three) are responsible for daily cleaning of the hospital facilities.
2. *Cleaning Staff Changes:* Job descriptions, policies and procedures, personnel assignments, and scheduling of work were all updated immediately by hospital administration and the new director of the department. In addition, all employees were interviewed regarding past performance, attitudes, and ideas for improvement. This resulted in replacement of approximately 25 percent of the cleaning personnel. Primary reasons for replacement included personnel unqualified for the job, poor attitude, and poor attendance.
3. *Training Program Changes:* The department now provides training for all employees on an ongoing basis:
   a. Training of new and current employees is provided on the job and in regularly scheduled sessions. Typical training session subjects include discharge cleaning, isolation cleaning, daily patient room cleaning, office and floor care cleaning, and informal sensitivity training.

b. Regular staff meetings are conducted to keep employees informed and to allow their input. Guest lectures are provided with representatives from other departments.

4. *Clean Equipment:* A total equipment replacement program was put into effect and was fully implemented within six months. This involved special training sessions for employees on proper use and maintenance of the equipment.

5. *Quality Control:* A complete revision of the former program has taken place. The revised program includes several major components:

   a. *Objectivity:* The areas selected for inspection are chosen randomly. The director of the program and his assistant perform all inspections. The standards are rigid and result in either a "satisfactory" or an "unsatisfactory" rating.

   b. *Accountability:* The hospital is divided into four major areas, with a supervisor responsible for each area. Each supervisor is responsible for the quality of service within his area. The results are used as a major factor in evaluating the employees' overall performance.

   c. *Incentives:* Quality indexes, by area and by supervisor, are posted weekly in the department to create interest and initiative on the part of the supervisors. In addition, an employee award program has been established for the cleaning staff. This has resulted in increased interest and positive competition throughout the program.

6. *Controls:* The program is controlled through feedback in the form of reports. Detailed reports are provided to supervisors for review with the cleaning staff. These reports provide specific information on areas inspected and, most importantly, indicate where improvement is required. Additional reports are generated for the hospital administration and for the director of the program.

Results of the program have been very significant. It was determined prior to implementation of the program that the overall quality of the facility was approximately 70 percent out of a possible 100 percent. A goal of 90 percent was set for achievement within six months.

Program results for the first three months of the program were 84 percent, 87 percent, and 88 percent respectively. Because of these favorable results, a decision was made to assign a "minimum" quality level of 80 percent and a "desirable" quality level of 95 percent.

After six months the program was regularly producing results within these control limits and the limits have now been changed to 85 percent (minimum) and 95 percent (desired). The program to date has been producing consistently within these limits.

*Conclusion*

Good leadership and proper management systems and controls are basic components for the provision of quality services and for employee job satisfaction. The basic requirements for employees at all levels is to know what is expected of them, to be provided with the proper tools, and to be rewarded appropriately for jobs well done. This reduces ambiguity, conflict, and counterproductive behavior, and thus reduces necessary management time.

The ultimate responsibility for allowing a situation to deteriorate in the manner described above lies with the hospital administration. The only way for top management to effectively produce high quality of services on an ongoing basis is to: (1) establish effective programs at the outset, (2) maintain and update the programs through feedback controls, and (3) maintain a continuous working relationship with department heads and other members of middle management.

The housekeeping department operations at this community hospital have been rehabilitated successfully, primarily because the above criteria are being met. Current operations are efficient, effective, and managed properly in terms of controls and use of time.

## PHYSICIAN PRODUCTIVITY

Most of the data, research, and experiences presented in this book focus upon the health care administrator and not the provider himself. Yet the discussion of productivity would not be complete without some commentary regarding the activities of the physician. Figure 5-7 presents the weekly number of patients seen in office, home, and hospital by active physicians engaged in private practice (by age of physician). Data collected in 1969 are compared with those from a 1942 study of the same nature. What is interesting to note is that the greatest amount of time is required of physicians between the ages of 30 to 40, a period when stress is at a peak as individuals perceive their lives and careers to be on a descending path. The high death rate between 35 and 40 may be attributable to the shock following this realization (Jacques, 1973, p. 154). The shock also often creates a period of depression, which increases the individual's vulnerability to stress-induced illness (Appelbaum, 1980, p. 10). It appears that this peak of productivity may be interrupted by unknown factors which reduce efficiency and loss of valuable time.

**Figure 5-7** Number of Patients Seen in Private Practice: A Contrast of Years and Physician Age

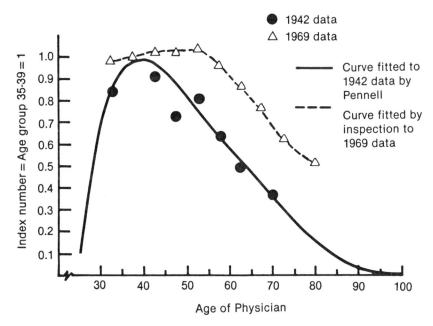

*Source:* Pennell, 1944, pp. 290-298, and Balfe, et al., 1971, p. 59. Reprinted with the permission of the American Medical Association.

We have other data with regard to physician productivity and time commitments. Table 5-2 presents data collected from an American Medical Association study that compares workload in terms of service per week and per hour of direct care among general practitioners, internists, and pediatricians. The results suggest that general practitioners are more productive in direct care than internists, with the differences being greatest in metropolitan areas.

Other measures of input and productivity can be studied by examining the size of organization within which the physician works. Table 5-3 presents the results of a study of a sample of internists. In this study, office visits are weighted by assigning to the major categories of regular office visits, annual examinations and complete histories and physical examinations, weights based upon the amount of time the physician normally devotes to each service output. Although physicians in larger partnerships and groups are supplemented to a greater degree by the services of other personnel, their productivity in terms of office visits is not increased. What is increased is income.

**Table 5-2** Specified Measures of Workload and Productivity by Selected Specialty, Sample of Physicians, U.S.A., 1969

| Specialty | Weeks Worked Per Year | Hours Worked Per Week | Hours of Direct Care Per Week | Visits Per Week | | | Total Visits Per Hour of Direct Care |
|---|---|---|---|---|---|---|---|
| | | | | Total | Office | Hospital | |
| General practice | 48.3 | 52.0 | 47.8 | 167.0 | 129.5 | 28.2 | 3.49 |
| Internal medicine | 47.9 | 52.8 | 47.7 | 127.2 | 86.3 | 33.5 | 2.67 |
| Pediatrics | 48.1 | 52.9 | 46.9 | 146.5 | 125.3 | 19.0 | 3.12 |

*Source:* Balfe, Lorant, and Todd, 1971, pp. 50-54. Reprinted with the permission of the American Medical Association.

**Table 5-3** Measures of Input and of Production, by Size of Organization

| Measures of Input and Output | Solo (N=12) | 2-man (N=4) | 3-man (N=6) | 4 to 5-man (N=5) | Clinics (N=4) |
|---|---|---|---|---|---|
| *Input measures* | | | | | |
| Average hours per physician | 218 | 222 | 197 | 200 | 197 |
| Average paramedical hours per physician | 187 | 181 | 225 | 271 | 499 |
| Average technical hours per physician | 7 | 11 | 9 | 44 | 122 |
| Average paramedical hours per physician hour | 0.858 | 0.817 | 1.142 | 1.353 | 2.531 |
| Average technical hours per physician hour | 0.032 | 0.050 | 0.046 | 0.220 | 0.619 |
| *Output (production) measures* | | | | | |
| Office visits per physician | 286 | 278 | 291 | 243 | 286 |
| Office visits per physician time with patients | 3.4 | 3.0 | 3.5 | 3.1 | 2.9 |
| Gross monthly income per physician | $4,777 | — | $6,107 | — | $6,725 |
| Average percent of revenues earned by sale of ancillary products | 15% | — | 34% | — | 48% |

*Source:* R.M. Bailey, "Economies of Scale in Medical Practice." In H.E. Klarman (Ed.), *Empirical Studies in Health Economics,* 1970. Used by permission of the Johns Hopkins University Press.

Another study of time worked, productivity, income, and quality of care was conducted in Canada and found that physicians in group practice work longer hours in Ontario than in Nova Scotia and earn more per hour of work. The differences in quality of care that appear to be a bit more for group practice are not significant. These data are presented in Table 5-4.

Another study (Yankauer et al., 1970) examined delegation and productivity in group practice. This focused on the utilization of auxiliary personnel and the propensity to delegate activities to such personnel as factors in the productivity of physicians in different types of practice.

The study reported findings from a mailed questionnaire survey of 90 percent of board certified pediatricians who graduated from medical schools after 1930. Productivity was viewed in terms of median hours spent in the office per week,

**Table 5-4** Hours of Work, Quality of Care, and Hourly Median Net Professional Income, by Type of Practice, Samples of General Practitioners

| Inputs and Outputs | Ontario | Nova Scotia |
|---|---|---|
| Hours of work per week | | |
| Solo practice | 44.6 | — |
| Group of two or more | 68.2 | — |
| Quality of care, mean score | | |
| Solo practice (29, 28) | 54.6 | 42.4 |
| Group of two or more | 62.8 | 46.2 |
| Median net professional income per hour of work, in dollars | | |
| Solo practice | | |
| Without nursing or secretarial assistance (9, 11) | $4.19 | $3.24 |
| With nursing or secretarial assistance (19, 12) | 5.17 | 4.57 |
| Group of two (8, 4) | 6.09 | 4.99 |
| Group of more than two, with assistance (6, 8) | 8.17 | 4.29 |

*Source:* F. Clute, "Arrangements for Practice: Time and Content of the General Practitioner's Work." In *The General Practitioner: A Study of Medical Education and Practice in Ontario and Nova Scotia,* 1963, pp. 103, 318, 194. Used by permission of the University of Toronto Press.

---

median total visits per week, and a ratio of the second measure to the first, which gives a rough measure of visits per unit time. All these measures of production tended to show increases with number of physicians and number of other health workers per practice, and with the propensity to delegate tasks to persons other than the physician. The presence of at least one registered nurse among these persons had a significant enhancing effect on task delegation and production.

The effect of differences in case mix was also evident. The production of visits was negatively related to percent of cases that were for health supervision (as distinct from the care of illness), and the percent of health supervision visits that lasted 15 minutes or more. Contrary to expectation, the category of multispecialty groups (those with five or more physicians and five or more other health workers of whom at least one was a registered nurse) was not the most productive in terms of the indicators used.

Table 5-5 shows selected findings from this study, which document the relationships described above. To a degree these findings support the views and findings of Bailey (1970) shown in Table 5-3. Other research indicates that task delegation, hours of work, and the pace of work were influenced not so much by "administrative theory or organizational opportunity," as by demand (Donabedian, 1973, p. 314).

**Table 5-5**  Aspects of the Practice of Board-Certified Pediatricians, by Type of Practice and Number of Other Health Workers Employed

| Aspects of Practice | Solo Practice, Employing Additional Workers as Indicated Below | | | | Multispecialty Group Practice |
|---|---|---|---|---|---|
| | One Non-R.N. | One R.N. | Two Includes R.N. | Three Includes R.N. | |
| Median hours in office | 31.0 | 33.4 | 35.0 | 36.7 | 37.3 |
| Median total visits | 81.5 | 93.1 | 108.5 | 131.1 | 105.1 |
| Median total visits divided by median hours in office | 2.60 | 2.78 | 3.10 | 3.57 | 2.82 |
| Percent respondents delegating one or more tasks | 6.1 | 10.8 | 16.5 | 27.4 | 7.5 |
| Ratio of health supervision visits to illness visits | 1.5 | 1.2 | 1.1 | 0.9 | 0.7 |
| Percent of health supervision visits of 15 or more minutes | 76 | 68 | 57 | 52 | 63 |

*Source:* D. Yankauer, J.P. Connelly, and J.J. Feldman. "Physician Productivity in the Delivery of Ambulatory Care: Some Findings from a Survey of Pediatricians." *Medical Care,* Jan./Feb. 1970, pp. 34-40. Used by permission of publisher.

---

What is important in the productivity of physicians is not the size of their firm as measured by the quantity of physicians employed but the use of larger numbers of auxiliary personnel and the delegation to them of tasks usually performed by the physician. This approach achieves efficiency and effectiveness of time management.

## VALUE ANALYSIS

### A Better Way—At a Lower Cost, and in Time!

This chapter has presented a variety of management theories and techniques to help health care professionals become more productive and effective in the performance of their jobs. One more technique remains to be discussed—that of value analysis. This technique is most interesting and, because of its element of creativity, may also turn out to be the most self-satisfying and rewarding as well—especially for what Drucker has called the "Knowledge Workers," in contrast to manual workers (Drucker, 1968, p. 362). Yet it also has universal appeal and broad adaptability.

Simply stated, value analysis is a method of securing the same or better performance of a function or activity at a lesser total cost. Presented in another way, it means finding a better way to accomplish the desired end result. In Drucker's terms, we need to "work smarter." The term "value analysis" was coined in 1946 by Lawrence D. Miles who, as a manager for the General Electric Company, was primarily interested in using this concept to achieve lower manufacturing costs. He defined it as (1961, p. 1):

> . . . an organized creative approach which has for its purpose the efficient identification of unnecessary cost, i.e., cost which provides neither quality nor use nor life nor appearance nor customer features . . . (it) is *not* a substitute for conventional cost-reduction work methods. Rather, it is a patent and completely different procedure for accomplishing far greater results. It improves the effectiveness of work . . . it fills in blind spots.

One historic example of using value analysis is shipping goods in cardboard rather than wooden boxes in order to reduce weight and thus lower both the burden of handling and the cost of freight. Another common illustration is the use of cardboard or plastic milk containers rather than thick glass bottles (or cans), which were extremely heavy, had to be returned for reuse, and presented the additional hazard of personal injury.

Historically, value analysis has been an extremely constructive and useful tool for industrial management in achieving lower costs by fostering and promoting the use of less expensive materials and methods having at least equal or better performance characteristics. It does, however, demand an objective ongoing evaluation and review of innovative ideas, alternate procedures, and other changes that may produce positive results for workers, users of goods and services, and the organization itself. As a matter of practice, value analysis is often performed as a small group effort by those who are most familiar with the activity under examination.

Just as value analysis is a successful technique for reducing production and distribution costs, it can also provide a useful approach to more effective time management by identifying unnecessary or costly usage of time and recommending new and viable alternatives. Initially, attention should be focused on the performance of a specific function or activity as it is related to the use of time by one individual or a group of people. Beyond this, however, an analysis of how a possible change may directly or indirectly affect other elements of the organization is also of utmost importance. Value analysis can be examined and implemented in a most empirical manner using the problem-solving approach.

## Step One—Gather Data

The first step in conducting value analysis is to find out as much as possible about the particular duty or activity under scrutiny. Good, precise answers should be sought to questions such as the following:

1. What has to be done?
2. Who or what does it now?
3. What is its purpose?
4. How urgent is it?
5. How much time does it take?
6. What other people or activities are involved or affected?
7. Where is it done?
8. Is it necessary at all?

## Step Two—Use Imagination

Once quantifiable answers have been obtained, as many alternate solutions as possible should be offered and listed. This is the step in which an individual's imagination should be stretched. Each person participating should freely contribute ideas that have any bearing on the problem under consideration. Any possible innovation, even though seemingly impractical, should be mentioned and noted. To help in this process, some of the following questions may stimulate creative thinking:

1. Who else within the organization does or can do it?
2. Who else outside the organization does or can do it?
3. How else can this be done?
4. Can it be eliminated?
5. Can it be done more simply or in an easier way?
6. Can it be reduced in size or scope?
7. Does this duplicate any other activity?
8. What existing procedure can be substituted?
9. Can it be standardized?
10. Can it be done less frequently?
11. Where else do we do this?
12. Is this important for future activities?

## Step Three—Comparison

Each of the various alternatives or recommendations generated from step two are now subjected to "hard-nosed" appraisal, not just in terms of reducing or eliminating the present use of time, but also from the point of view of the total impact and cost in time on all aspects of the organization. Here the total value toward furthering or impeding the organization's objectives should be the criterion. Overall, and in the long run, what will be lost, or gained, by implementing this change? Finally, is the change really a desirable solution?

## Step Four—Buy It and Try It

After deciding on what seems to be the most promising and feasible alternative, the change should be initiated promptly and then, after a reasonable trial period, should be thoroughly assessed. If it is deemed that the adopted solution is not satisfactory, it should be adjusted, replaced by a second alternative, or completely abandoned in favor of returning to the original practice or procedure. This is actually the decision-making process in its total span of management effectiveness. In any case, there must be a valid rationale, justification, or positive result for instituting a change, and not merely the instituting of a change for the sake of change itself. The success or failure of change must be viewed not only in terms of one specific activity, but rather with regard to its effect on all other functions and components of the organization. It is quite conceivable that an effort to improve performance in one department may unsuspectingly trigger an excessive and costly expenditure of time in another. This is negative productivity, which is costly and time-consuming.

The remainder of this chapter will be devoted to describing a number of situations that illustrate the wide applicability of value analysis as a valuable tool for "knowledge workers" to use to achieve more production and more effective management of their own time, as well as that of their subordinates.

## Saving Someone Else's Time

Although value analysis is frequently conducted as a group or committee effort, an individual can successfully do it alone, as its purpose is seeking and finding practical improvements to specific problems or conditions.

## The Health Care Component

### Transfer Carts

One administrator explained how, by using value analysis, he was able to substantially reduce the size and value of his hospital's medication inventory. He did this by suggesting that the supply of all available and necessary medications, in specified patient areas, be contained and confined to a single medication transfer cart. He proposed a daily exchange with another one which was completely restocked. At first there was strong opposition because of the fear of a depleted inventory during an emergency situation, but after guaranteeing an extra 20 percent of all normally required pharmacy items, a trial was instituted. The outcome was an overall inventory reduction of 60 percent, as the previously mandated inventory size proved to be quite excessive. The final result was a much smaller investment in the hospital's total pharmacy product inventory and the release of some sorely needed storage space. With current escalating rates of inflation and the concomitant high cost of money, any means of achieving a reduction in the value of any inventory should be accorded the highest priority.

## Disposable Cups and Gowns

In this same institution, a change in the type and composition of a disposable drinking cup resulted in a savings of five cents per cup—in quantity, of course! And more recently, a careful analysis of the cost and maintenance of operating room gowns revealed that by substituting disposables, over $5,000 could be saved. The original idea for this change was submitted through a suggestion box, and the happy employee who made the recommendation received a personal bonus as a reinforcing mechanism.

## Security and Payroll

One hospital solved a couple of pressing problems by making its computer do the work. Each employee was provided with a plastic ID card capable of being recognized by strategically located electronic sensors tied in to the institution's computer. As an employee reported to work, the card was presented to a parking lot sensor. If parking in that lot was authorized, the barrier swung open and concurrently, for payroll purposes, the time of arrival was recorded in the computer's data bank. A similar procedure at the end of the work day dutifully noted the time of departure. Security within the building was controlled in like manner. Without the proper ID card, sensors denied access to restricted areas to all but previously authorized personnel. In effect, the computer performed functions which would otherwise have had to be accomplished by time clocks and payroll clerks, as well as a security staff charged with the responsibility of regulating parking and controlling the movement of people within the hospital. This is a fine example of higher productivity and reduced time involvement that adds to cost containment.

*Reports*

Health care institutions are certainly not immune from the deluge of information and escalating flow of paper which today seems to pervade all fields of organization. This is an excellent opportunity for practicing value analysis. The generation and the reading of proliferating numbers of reports, memoranda, letters, and other written material can, for many employees, become a most frustrating and time-consuming experience, to say nothing about the time required for duplication and distribution.

In conducting an investigation into the extent of the paper flow, the following questions should be helpful in establishing guidelines for reducing the size, scope, and frequency of reports and other written materials, particularly those of a recurring nature:

1. Why is the information needed?
2. Who needs the report?
3. Who wants the report? Why?
4. Is it comprehensive enough?
5. Is it too comprehensive?
6. Who receives copies?
7. Can the material be better presented in another form?
8. How frequently is the report prepared?
9. How many copies are distributed?
10. Can the report be combined with another report?
11. If the report were eliminated what would happen?
12. What other reports presently contain this information?
13. Must this information be considered a permanent record?
14. How can the report be improved?
15. Can this information be made available from the computer's data bank?
16. Who receives the report but doesn't really need it?

In appraising the significance, usefulness, and real need for various kinds of written data, i.e., statistical studies, memoranda, evaluations, and projections, special consideration should also be given to the cost, in time, of securing the raw data. This usually involves many people who may spend endless hours (time which may be used for a more important immediate need), searching and arranging material for the person who actually writes the final report.

Unless the intention is to produce a broad-based document, like a house organ, to disseminate information or news in general, it is expedient to have prescribed definitive distribution patterns for specific kinds of data. This will inform those persons who need to be kept up to date and not waste the time and clutter the files of those who may find it irrelevant to their tasks.

# REFERENCES

American Hospital Association. *The management of hospital employee productivity: An introductory handbook.* Chicago: American Hospital Association, 1973.

Ammer, D.S. *Materials management* (Rev. ed.). Homewood, Ill.: Richard D. Irwin Co., 1968.

Appelbaum, S.H. Managerial/organizational stress: Identification of factors and symptoms. *Health Care Management Review,* Winter 1980, 5(1).

Bailey, R.M. Economies of scale in medical practice. In H.E. Klarman (Ed.), *Empirical studies in health economics.* Baltimore: Johns Hopkins Press, 1970.

Balfe, B.E., Lorant, J.H., & Todd, C. *Reference data on the profile of medical practice 1971.* Chicago: Center for Health Services Research and Development, American Medical Association, 1971.

Bartscht, K.G. Summary status report on the development and implementation of an innovative quality-producing management program. Ann Arbor: Chi Systems, Inc., 1978.

Becker, S.W., & Neuhauser, D. *The efficient organization.* New York: Elsevier Publishing, 1975.

Bennett, A.C. *Improving management performance in health care institutions: A total systems approach.* Chicago: American Hospital Association, 1978.

Clute, F. Arrangements for practice: Time and content of the general practitioner's work. In *The general practitioner: A study of medical education and practice in Ontario and Nova Scotia.* Toronto: University of Toronto Press, 1963.

Dobbs, C.E. Improving productivity: Ways to get people started. *Supervisory Management,* March 1976, *21,* 2-6.

Donabedian, A. *Aspects of medical care administration: Specifying requirements for health care.* Cambridge, Mass.: Harvard University Press, 1973.

Drucker, P. *The age of discontinuity.* New York: Harper and Row, 1968.

Ganett, W.J. Production and operations management. New York: Harcourt Brace and World, 1968.

Garbarino, J.W. Some demand and supply considerations. In *Health Plans and Collective Bargaining.* Berkeley: University of California Press, 1960.

Hayes, D.A. The evaluation of management. *Financial Analysts Journal,* July-August 1968, *24.*

Jacques, E. *Work, creativity and social justice.* New York: International Universities Press, 1973.

Johnson, E.A. Physician productivity and the hospital: A hospital administrator's view. *Inquiry,* September 1969, *6,* 59-69.

Malcolm, J. & Rowe, A.J. (Eds.). *A symposium on management information and control systems: Management control systems.* New York: Wiley, 1960.

Miles, L.D. *Techniques of value analysis and engineering.* New York: McGraw-Hill Book Co., 1961.

Misumi, J., & Shirakashi, S. An experimental study of the effects of supervisory behavior on productivity and morale in a hierarchical organization. *Human Relations,* 1966, *19.*

Pennell, E.H. Location and movement of physicians—methods for estimating physician resources. *Public Health Reports.* March 3, 1944, *59,* 281-305.

Rutstein, D.R. *Blueprint for medical care.* Cambridge, Mass., MIT Press, 1974.

Sayles, L.R. Managing human resources for higher productivity. *The Conference Board Record,* July 1973, *10.*

Wofford, J.C. Managerial behavior, situational factors, and productivity and morale. *Administrative Science Quarterly,* March 1971, *16.*

Wolfe, S., Badgley, R.F., Kasius, R.V., Garson, J.Z., & Gold, R.J.M. The work of a group of doctors in Saskatchewgn. *Milbank Memorial Fund Quarterly*, January 1968, *46*, 103-129.

Yankauer, D., Connelly, J.P., & Feldman, J.J. Physician productivity in the delivery of ambulatory care: Some findings from a survey of pediatricians. *Medical Care*, January-February 1970, *8*, 35-46.

# Chapter 6

# Managerial Roles of Health Care Administrators

**TIME MANAGEMENT HIGHLIGHTS**

1. Changes that have occurred in hospital administration in the past ten years include the increasing complexity of medical care, the increasing extent of external controls on the hospital, and the change in public expectations toward more extensive services and better health care from the system as a whole. Due to the increased responsibilities of health care administrators, the chief executive officer must delegate more of his authority and no longer can be in daily contact with most of the issues facing the hospital.

2. Chief executive officers of smaller institutions engage in fewer formal activities but are much more concerned with the operating work of their organizations.

3. Health care executives spend a high percentage of time alone and with administrative subordinates. They spend a small amount of time with medical personnel, patients, and board members. Conversations occupy over 60 percent of their time, while observing and thinking alone occupy relatively little time.

4. A study of chief executives found no break in the pace of activity during office hours. The mail, phone, and meetings accounted for almost every minute from the moment these men entered their offices in the morning until they departed in the evening.

5. The question of why these managers adopt this pace and workload can be explored by examining the openended nature of their jobs. They are responsible for the success of their organization and there are no tangible mileposts where they can stop and realize their job is finished.

6. Half of their activities are completed in less than nine minutes and managers are not willing to spend much time on any one issue in any one session. In addition, managers frequently interrupt their desk work to place phone calls or request subordinates to drop in. The manager tolerates interruptions because he does not wish to discourage the flow of current information.

7. The manager is encouraged by the realities of his work to develop a particular personality—to overload himself with work, to do things abruptly, to avoid wasting time, to participate only when the value of participation is tangible, to avoid too great an involvement with any one issue. We may characterize the manager's position as the neck of an hourglass. He sits between the network of contacts and his organization, sifting what is received from the outside and sending much of it into his organization.

8. There are eight managerial types:

   a. contact man              e. real-time manager
   b. political manager        f. team manager
   c. entrepreneur             g. expert manager
   d. insider                  h. new manager

9. The manager's time assumes an enormous opportunity cost. Lacking time, he can inhibit organizational development by postponing requests for authorization, by delaying improvement projects, by reducing the amount of information he disseminates, and so on.

10. By bringing more consistency to the manager's scheduled activity, by relieving him of much of the need to schedule his own work, and by using systematic analysis to design his schedule in accordance with his needs and those of his health care organization, the management technologist can actualize greater gains in efficiency and effectiveness.

Changes that have occurred in hospital administration in the last ten years include the increasing complexity of medical care, the increasing extent of external controls on the hospital, and the change in public expectations toward better and more extensive services from the health care system as a whole. The change in the role of the health care administrator toward much broader responsibility and greatly increased complexity has been clear. Outside interests were formerly responsible for controlling many hospital decisions, which removed many management prerogatives from the health care administrator.

A major change in the administrative role is that success is no longer generally defined as merely increasing the size and scope of a hospital's services. In fact, some administrators indicate that effectiveness of services and more cost-efficient delivery of services may very well be the critical marks of administrator success.

A decrease in flexibility has been emphasized as a recent critical change. Government purchase of services and governmental planning activities definitely constrain the hospital administrator's ability to act in what might be his most preferred mode. In fact, most of the changes identified in the recent ten years have been due to external forces. The chief executive officer has become more involved in external contacts and has become an external strategist for dealing with his organization's environment.

Perhaps one major favorable outcome of these changes has been a movement away from a crisis-oriented, firefighting type of administration toward a more carefully developed long-range planning format in many institutions. Recent trends in governmental regulations seems to indicate that this shift toward planning will now be combined with regulatory determinations by planning agencies.

## CHANGING ROLES

The present role of these administrators is changing, however. In general, given the increased external pressures on hospital administrators and on hospitals in recent years, one would expect that the present role of the hospital administrator would be fairly difficult and demanding. Such appears to be the case. One administrator made the comment, somewhat facetiously, that the problems facing the hospital today are sufficiently stringent that any discussion of the future role of hospital administrators would have to wait until he had time for it (Forrest, Johnson, & Mosher, 1976, p. 435).

Due to the increased responsibilities of health care administrators, the chief executive officer must delegate more of his authority and no longer can be in daily contact with most of the issues facing the hospital. Many hospital administrators are adopting a role division of internal operating officer and external contact person. Without this role division, the administrator has tremendous demands on his time which result in problems such as not having the time to keep on top of what is occurring at all levels of the hospital or dealing only with high-priority issues.

When we speak about administering in the field of health care medicine, we refer to those nontechnical activities that should be performed by the leader of the department. Ideally, the leader should be a physician. However, the role is tied not to the M.D. degree, but to a function, namely, that of organizing and coordinating the activities of a varied number of health personnel through cooperative means and direct action toward the attainment of a common goal.

To manage, one must be able to control. Consequently, the manager must know what authority he possesses to perform his function. Thus the manager will make decisions the nature of which will be affected by the demands of the environment, the institution, and his particular department. In that role he will be acting as the leader and should be using his decision-making powers in accordance with the overall management policy of the hospital. To achieve his goal he must set objectives, both short- and long-term. A subfunction of objective setting is the constraint to be realistic. The objectives should have reasonable time limits for their completion and should be measurable, specific, and attainable (Yanda, 1977, p. 29).

The concept of administering and authority are intricately interwoven. Chester Barnard (1968, p. 163) has developed the most insightful definition of authority.

> Authority is the character of a communication (order) in a formal organization by virtue of which it is accepted by a contributor to or "member" of the organization as governing the action he contributes; that is, as governing or determining what he does or is not to do so far as the organization is concerned. According to this definition, authority involves two aspects: first, the subjective, and personal—the accepting of a communication as authoritative, and, second, the objective—the character in the communication by virtue of which it is accepted.

If a directive is accepted by one to whom it is addressed, its authority for him is confirmed or established. Disobedience of such a communication is a denial of its authority for him. Therefore, under this definition the decision as to whether an order has authority or not lies with the persons to whom it is addressed and does not reside in persons of authority or those who issue the orders.

The utilization of authority and assumption of the role of administrator is doubly conflicting and time-consuming for physicians who assume the position of administrator in a health care system within which they previously functioned in a technical manner. As individuals, physicians have no problem in responding appropriately to stimuli for which they have been previously and appropriately conditioned. However, when the physician is confronted with situations for which no previous program exists, it will be his philosophical basis that will likely determine the nature and extent of his reaction. Thus the physician, never having been programmed to work as a manager or with a team, much less as a leader of it, is likely to run into situations that will require a response from him for which he has no established guidelines. This leads to additional investment in managerial resources and time.

The role of the health care manager as an interlocking resource within the system is crucial. It is as crucial for those individuals with business expertise as it is for medically trained administrators. These managers must juggle two interest groups (medical staff and physicians), which is usually accomplished through the vehicle of a committee—often thought of as a time-saving, decision-making body. This process, however, is not without problems.

The easiest way to destroy a hospital-based physician is to continually chip away at his requests in committees by delaying or sidetracking them for procedural reasons. Each delaying action is so minor that it is soon forgotten, except by the target of the action, but it has a cumulative effect. If a manager is to develop a reputation for effectiveness and success, it is imperative that the majority of committee requests be granted. In addition, successes must be highly visible to build up the reputation of the health care manager and increase inputs into the power circles.

The committee is the organizational unit of the hospital's medical staff structure. Its function is to receive input from a variety of members who then work out jointly accepted policies and develop plans appropriate for long-range targets. Although the implementation of those plans may be the prerogative of single individuals, development of and agreement on the plans inevitably requires group action. A more thorough enumeration of the functions of committees would include the following (Yanda, 1977, p. 119):

- To mutually educate the membership in the complexities of a given situation.

- To develop a consensus on an agreeable response in a complex situation.

- When alternative actions are possible, to choose the best one.

- To provide a meeting ground, with formal rules of conduct, for resolution of actual or potential conflicts among opposing points of view.

- To provide a forum for planning with additional input from less concerned areas.

- To coordinate the actions of one or more groups.

- To provide a formal setting for peer review or other judicial processes.

- To formally and openly review the qualifications of new applicants to the staff.

- To provide an effective means of communication with another organization, particularly one at a higher level. (In general, rigidly structured groups have great difficulty in communicating with an individual except insofar as he is a representative of another group. Therefore, if you wish to communicate with an organized group, especially at government level, it is best to invest your input with the same trappings.)

Administrators need a direct line to the power pockets of their hospital. If this is not the case, then all proposals will be subjected to committee approval throughout the decision-making process.

The departments of pathology, radiology, and anesthesiology may or may not have specific departmental committees, but they invariably have one important asset: the heads of their departments sit on the executive committee. The chief pathologist, radiologist, and anesthesiologist may not have votes on that committee, but their very presence gives them an additional power connection that other department heads do not have.

A list of some regular hospital medical staff committees includes:

- Executive Committee of the Medical Staff
- Joint Conference Committee—Executive Committee and Hospital Board representation
- Department of Medicine
- Department of Surgery
- Department of Family Practice
- Department of Pediatrics
- Department of Obstetrics and Gynecology
- Department of Anesthesia
- Department of Outpatient Services and Emergency Room
- Department of Radiology
- Department of Pathology and Laboratory Services
- Tissue and Transfusion Committee
- Utilization Review Committee
- Credentials Committee
- Critical Care Committee
- Infectious Disease Committee
- Continuing Medical Education Committee
- Patient Care Services Committee
- Medical Records Committee
- Library Committee
- Pharmacy Committee
- Medical Care Evaluation or Audit and Peer Review Committee

These committees may require the administrator to serve on several of them throughout his tenure.

The advantage of multiple committee assignments is the opportunity to choose the most suitable location for expounding new proposals and ideas. The disadvantage is that if your department is involved in more than one committee and you cannot be present at all of the meetings, you may be assured, by the principle of Murphy's law, that if something can go wrong, it will. It is in the one meeting you miss that your department will be discussed in far greater detail than you might have wished. Of course, that can also happen on committees of which you are not a member. If you have a structured department with a departmental supervisor appointed by the hospital, it is useful to make his availability known to all committee chairmen. Thus if questions arise and you are not available to answer them, the questioners have someone else to approach.

You may also request that the supervisor be allowed to attend meetings when you are not available, not only to provide necessary departmental input but also to receive feedback that might modify departmental activities. Unfortunately, physicians on the whole prefer not to have nonphysicians at their meetings, owing to the delicate matters that they sometimes discuss in a rather spontaneous fashion. It is increasingly common for administrative personnel to be at major committee meetings, but it would be political to get approval before you have your assistant stand in for you (Yanda, 1977, p. 122).

Some of these suggestions are worthy of consideration from an efficient time use perspective. The literature of management contains many references to time conservation, to the use of time and motion studies, and to the improvement of executive performance. Paradoxically, however, relatively few empirical studies provide any direct linkage between work patterns of executives and administrators and how they use their time.

In *The Effective Executive* Peter Drucker (1967, p. 35) notes that interest in measuring and evaluating the use of time has largely been confined to unskilled and skilled manual work. In expanding on this idea, he states:

> We have applied this knowledge for the work where time does not greatly matter, that is, where the difference between time-use and time-waste is primarily efficiency and costs. But we have not applied it to the work that matters increasingly, and particularly has to cope with time: the work of the knowledge worker and especially the executive. Here the difference between time-use and time-waste is effectiveness and results.

In commenting on future aspects of managerial work, Henry Mintzberg (1973, pp. 197-198) calls for better job descriptions, more and diversified research, and greater interest in the study of job differences. He concludes:

Considering the upsurge in management research in the last decade, it is surprising that managerial work has received so little attention. . . . We can no longer afford to ignore managerial work as an area of research. It is the researcher, feeding knowledge to the manager and management scientist, who will ultimately determine the ability of our large bureaucracies to cope with their immense problems.

## A HISTORIC VIEW OF THE WORLD OF THE MANAGER

For the purpose of providing some background material for comparative purposes, a brief review of some prior studies is presented.

While early writings in the field of management indicate a strong interest in how time is used, this interest was particularly centered on those performing manual work. In *The Principles of Scientific Management,* Frederick Taylor (1911, p. 30) introduced the "task idea" as one of the basic elements of scientific management. In this concept he included first, what is to be accomplished, and second, the exact amount of time allowed for its completion. Concern for the physical aspects of work was continued by Frank and Lillian Gilbreth who conducted motion studies and designed devices and procedures specifically to reduce fatigue. Throughout their work they showed a keen awareness for a common and universal constraint—time—in regard to promoting greater worker productivity.

The work of the executive has been the focus and impetus of much research. In the early 1930's Luther Gulick asked the question: "What is the work of the chief executive? What does he do?" The answer is POSDCORB.

POSDCORB is, of course, a made-up word designed to call attention to the various functional elements of the work of a chief executive because "administration" and "management" have lost all specific content. POSDCORB is made up of the initials of and stands for the following activities:

1. *Planning*—working out in broad outline the things that need to be done and the methods for doing them to accomplish the purpose set for the enterprise;
2. *Organizing*—establishing the formal structure of authority through which work subdivisions are arranged, defined, and coordinated for the defined objective;
3. *Staffing*—the personnel function of bringing in and training staff and maintaining favorable conditions of work;
4. *Directing*—the continuous task of making decisions and embodying them in specific and general orders and instruction and serving as the leader of the enterprise;
5. *Coordinating*—the all-important duty of interrelating the various parts of the work;

6. *Reporting*—keeping those to whom the executive is responsible informed as to what is going on, which includes keeping himself and his subordinates informed through records, research, and inspection;

7. *Budgeting*—fiscal planning, accounting, and control.

This statement of the work of a chief executive is interpreted from the functional analysis elaborated by Henri Fayol in his *Industrial and General Administration* (Gulick and Urwick, 1973). It is believed that those who know administration intimately will find in this analysis a valid and helpful pattern, into which can be fitted each of the major activities and duties of any chief executive (Gulick and Urwick, 1973, p. 13).

One of the first studies to indicate a shift of attention away from manual workers and toward top management was published in 1951 by Sune Carlson. Following Barnard's suggestion of five bases of specialization—place, time, persons, things, and method of process (Barnard, 1978, pp. 128-129), and using a log reporting form, Carlson explored the time use of nine top-level Swedish businessmen, looking for common patterns and relationships that would characterize their work. Carlson found that his executives spent little time alone in their offices, with much time devoted to conferences and visits. Forty percent of their time was spent outside the firm. Carlson identified the following problem areas (1951, pp. 62-64):

1. Activities outside the firm.
2. Lack of time for inspecting and visiting works and offices.
3. Lack of time for reading and contemplation.
4. The excessive nature of the total workload.

Carlson analyzed the place of work, the technique of communication, and the total workload. Best known is his finding about the rarity of uninterrupted time. Citing one example, Carlson indicated that although executives averaged about one hour alone each day, the typical "alone" intervals were of only 10 to 15 minutes duration, and only 12 times during the 35 days were they alone for more than 22 minutes. "All they knew was that they scarcely had time to start on a new task or to sit down and light a cigarette before they were interrupted by a visitor or a telephone call" (Carlson, 1951, pp. 73-74). Carlson felt that managers could easily lengthen the average duration of their tasks and avoid fragmentation and interruption. This could be accomplished by delegating more to clerical help. One must question at this point whether managers actually avoid fragmentation or seek it out. Carlson also concluded that the executives' workloads were heavy, averaging between 8.5 and 11.5 hours daily, which precluded significant social and cultural activity. He noted that the executives had little control over the design of their own workdays (Mintzberg, 1973, p. 203).

In 1954 Tom Burns, following Carlson's initial impetus, studied four employees in middle management positions in a British engineering firm. The longest time use he found was in conversation, 80 percent, with the remaining time spent reading or writing alone (Burns, 1954, p. 78). A few years later Burns reported his findings of 76 top management people. He concluded (1957, p. 48): "Heads of concerns, or their immediate deputies in some cases, worked much longer hours than most. . . . Executives with fairly defined functions—accountants, senior draughtsmen, production controllers—worked least hours." Because of the large amount of time top-level managers spent talking to one another, and the small amount of time spent with subordinates, Burns suggests (1957, p. 60):

> The accepted view of management as a working hierarchy on organizational chart lines may be dangerously misleading. Management simply does not operate as a flow of information up through a succession of filters, and a flow of decisions and instructions down through a succession of amplifiers.

In 1963 three Europeans, Copeman, Luijk, and Hanika conducted independent time studies of executives and made these observations (1963, pp. 120-121):

1. Increased attention to executives' time use will influence future layouts of office buildings.
2. Control information requires wider distribution so that executives may monitor their own time use.
3. Senior executives should engage in continuous learning and teaching.
4. A senior executive can allocate his time better if he knows where in his firm the source of main flow of ideas is located.

Copeman actually used a diary to contrast the work of 29 chief executives with a similar number of department heads. He found that the chief executives spent more time on the job (53 versus 43 hours per week) and more time "writing" and "planning," but less time drafting reports. The frequency of their contacts with subordinates was the same as for the department heads, but they had fewer with superiors (1.5 percent versus 14.5 percent) and more with their colleagues (16 percent versus 10.5 percent).

Horne and Lupton (1965) surveyed industrial middle managers in 1965 in order to investigate various patterns of activity as a basis for designing, administering, and teaching courses of study for managers and candidates for managerial positions. From a sample of 66 they concluded that their subjects spent most of their time during the work week ". . . creating, collecting, assembling, integrating, and regulating the necessary resources. They do not spend much time policy-making and planning" (p. 25). They concluded that these individuals were not overworked and that the time spent in particular functional areas indicated specialization by type of manager but not by level. The managers spent most of their time on nonformulating activities.

Miriam Dolson summarized the findings of a Cornell University pilot study of "How Hospital Administrators Rate Different Tasks" in the June 1965 issue of *Modern Hospital*. This research was designed primarily to ascertain the relative importance administrators attach to selected problem areas. By ranking specified problems by "demand time," approximately 200 responses rated the following as first to fourth in importance:

- Department heads
- Business and finance
- Personnel management
- Medical staff
- Planning and patient care
- Community relations
- Governing board
- Physical plant
- Problems of control
- Legal aspects

Rosemary Stewart investigated how 160 British managers used their time, and published her comprehensive findings in 1967 (pp. 101-127). Using a log reporting form somewhat like Carlson's, she also wanted answers to when, where, what, how, and with whom. By averaging time use and using a specially designed computer software package, she identified five distinct job types:

1. Emissaries, who spend much of their time outside the firm.
2. Writers or specialist managers, who work much of the time by themselves.
3. Discussers, who use a lot of time talking and listening in an effort to get other people to do something.
4. Trouble shooters, who have a fragmented work pattern.
5. Committee men, who use a lot of time in group discussions and have a wide range of contacts.

In analyzing her data, Stewart notes that apart from a specified function, such as sales or production, which affects how a manager uses his time, three other factors were relevant (1967, pp. 136-138):

1. The extent of involvement with the general management of the firm.
2. Number of employees.
3. The way in which the firm was organized.

Some of the main findings of this study are:

- The managers averaged 42 hours of work per week.

- 75 percent of their time was spent in their own establishment and 51 percent in their own offices.

- 60 percent of their time was spent in discussion—43 percent informal, 7 percent committee, 6 percent telephoning, and 4 percent social activity.

- 34 percent of their time was spent alone, 25 percent with their immediate subordinates, 8 percent with their superiors, and 30 percent with peers and others (of this, 12 percent with colleagues reporting to the same superior, 8 percent with those doing similar work elsewhere in the organization, 5 percent with other internal contacts, and 5 percent with external contacts).

- Fragmentation of work was great, according to each of three measures: in four weeks, the managers averaged only nine periods of 30 minutes or more without interruption (and four out of five managers had fewer than 15 such periods); the managers averaged 12 fleeting contacts per day (i.e., less than 5 minutes duration); they averaged another 13 diary entries per day, for a total of 25.

- "A manager's job is a varied one . . . in the place of work, in the contacts, in its activities and in its content" (p. 98).

A summary of her findings offers the opportunity for a number of interesting comparisons:

1. Few managers worked long hours.
2. Most managers spent some time outside the firm.
3. Discussion used more than half of the managers' time.
4. Managers who were concerned with problems outside their own department spent more time in discussion and less on paperwork and inspection.
5. On the average, respondents were with people two thirds of the time and size of firm was a factor in using time for discussion.
6. Time used for single and group discussions was equally divided, with immediate subordinates taking most of it.
7. It is possible to distinguish differences between managers' jobs on the basis of time use. The jobs can also be classified into groups on this basis.

8. The main difference between groups is the type of job and the function performed.
9. There is a tendency for contact time to increase with the number of employees.

In 1968 the St. Louis University Program in Hospital Administration conducted a time study of top administrators in Catholic and non-Catholic hospitals. The following were part of the general conclusions (Murray et al., 1968, p. 49):

• Administrators of the 300-399 bed-size and larger facilities, both Catholic and non-Catholic, spent a greater proportion of their time interacting with mixed groups at various levels.

• The greatest amount of time spent with administrative staff is by administrators of the larger (300+ bed) hospitals, both Catholic and non-Catholic.

• Administrators of non-Catholic hospitals allocate a greater proportion of their time to medical staff interactions with those in the larger (300+ bed) hospitals allocating approximately 10 percent.

"Toward More Effective Management," a study by The United Hospital Fund of New York (p. 17), was published in 1973. The primary aim of this research was to examine the development of better health care managers. Interviews and questionnaires were used to evaluate the validity of seven basic requirements of an "effective manager" in terms of individual performance, overall institutional operation, and the individual's training and development efforts. To an openended question which probed for barriers that precluded the attainment of the stated requirements, both "absence of training" and "time constraints and work pressures" ranked within the top five reasons offered by respondents.

Henry Mintzberg's significant work on how managers spend their time appeared in 1973 in his text *The Nature of Managerial Work*. He sought answers to "What do managers do?" by conducting intensive personal observations of five executives, one of whom was a hospital administrator. From his study he identified six sets of characteristics and ten basic managerial roles. From his analysis, Mintzberg suggests a contingency theory that attributes differences and variations to environmental, job, personal, and situational variables. He supports Stewart's findings concerning organizational size (1973, p. 104):

The size of the overall organization appears to have a considerable effect on what its senior managers do. . . . The chief executives of smaller organizations engage in fewer formal activities but are much more concerned with the operating work of their organizations.

In commenting about differences between business firms and public organizations, he says that the latter ". . . faced more complex coalitions of external forces—the chief executive spent more time in formal activity and more time meeting with outside groups, clients and directors" (1973, p. 108). Mintzberg further notes that successful managers (p. 125):

> . . . are likely to demonstrate a special ability to operate in peer relationships, to lead others in subordinate relationships, to resolve interpersonal and decisional conflicts, to deal in the verbal media, to make complex interrelated decisions, to allocate resources (including their own time), and to innovate.

Mintzberg studied the activities of a health care manager and found that due to the particularly high status in the field of medicine of both the hospital and its director, Manager C was required to interact frequently with peers and trade organizations (10 percent versus 1 percent of contacts). Many status requests and solicitations were made of him (11 percent versus 3 percent of verbal contacts) and a large number of trade publications were submitted to him for review (20 percent versus 5 percent of mail from trade organizations). No doubt all hospital administrators receive a large number of status requests from members of the communities they serve. Furthermore, there appears to be a well-developed communication system in the hospital community, particularly with regard to the distribution of medical reports. The prestige of Manager C and his hospital served to magnify these characteristics.

Furthermore, the internal workings of this organization (and no doubt, of hospitals in general) were characterized by a very high level of internal democracy. The professional staffers were highly trained, high-income individuals who conducted many of their affairs as they alone saw fit. In simple terms, there tended to be much internal "political" activity, and this influenced the chief executive's work. His unscheduled meetings were longer (24 versus 11 minutes on average) since people who dropped in had to be allowed to state their cases. As might further be expected in this milieu, the flow of documented information was lighter, while verbal information flowed more freely. Information related to organizational politics is seldom documented. Thus, there was in this organization a high frequency of meetings in the hall (7 percent versus 2 percent of contacts), a high frequency of two-person (tête-à-tête) scheduled meetings (61 percent versus 45 percent), a large proportion of Manager C's verbal contact time devoted to information processing (60 percent versus 34 percent), and little mail concerned with internal operations (8 percent versus 21 percent) (1973, p. 261).

## A CURRENT PERSPECTIVE ON THE WORK OF THE MANAGER

Information which reveals how a hospital chief executive officer uses time may not only prove valuable in evaluating his past performance, but also help to set criteria for future patterns, particularly in terms of Drucker's "systematic time management."

For the specific purpose of determining how individuals use their time, a study was conducted of 24 top-level nonmedical administrators in various sized hospitals in New Jersey and the metropolitan area of New York (Rohrs, 1979). All the employing institutions were classified as nongovernmental, short-term, general medical, and surgical by the American Hospital Association (1975). Each participant, a volunteer, was assured anonymity and was provided daily time log forms on which to record, by half-hour intervals, actual time use for a two-week period.

At this point it may be worthwhile to briefly consider some of the greatest difficulties in using a diary or log for reporting time use, particularly for measuring activity in terms of functions: planning, organizing, staffing, coordinating, and controlling. The basic problems are definition, interpretation, and, of course, overlap. In order to overcome these inherent difficulties, this study measured job characteristics rather than functions of work content. Mintzberg clearly delineates between these two approaches. "Characteristics" are defined as referring to questions of when, where, with whom, and how, whereas "categorizations of work content and purpose lead to statements of *functions* or *roles*" (1973, pp. 223-224). This, of course, follows Barnard's suggestion mentioned earlier. Thus, in this particular research, only work characteristics were measured.

Another problem that may occur with using logs is the possibility of omitting or blurring short intervals of time. In an attempt to reduce these occurrences, this log included space for recording fragmented time periods, which were not otherwise indicated.

In this study, respondents reported their time use in terms of the following work characteristics: when (time interval), where (inside or outside of hospital); with whom (alone, with administrative colleague, administrative subordinate, board member, medical personnel, or patient, and other); and how (paperwork, conversing, observing, and thinking alone). In addition to providing space for noting fragmented time, another column was included for entering optional comments or explanatory remarks related to a particular event or special time use. Participants were encouraged to add extra time periods before and after the usual work day or week as necessary. The definitions of terms used are listed in Table 6-1.

Table 6-2 indicates summaries of ranges, means, and standard deviations of the work characteristics investigated, expressed as percentages of actual reported time. Table 6-3 provides similar information, but in actual recorded hours rather than in percentages.

**Table 6-1** Definitions

( 1) Administrative Colleague — Fellow hospital administrator in another hospital.

( 2) Administrative Subordinate — Nonmedical employee of hospital who is subject to supervision by respondent.

( 3) Board Member — Member(s) of the hospital's governing board.

( 4) Community Member — Outsiders from business, educational, social, religious, and social service organizations. Consultants and the press.

( 5) Medical Personnel — All medical personnel.

( 6) Patient — Person(s) admitted for treatment and/or observations.

( 7) Other — Person(s) not otherwise specified.

( 8) Paperwork — Reading, writing, numerical calculations. Preparing reports, correspondence.

( 9) Conversing — Face-to-face and telephone discussion with others for exchange of information and opinion. Interviewing. Giving instruction and direction.

(10) Observing — Visual observation of performance or behavior of people, procedures, or equipment.

(11) Thinking *Alone* — Problem solving, deliberation for evaluation and/or making a decision.

(12) Fragment — Time period characterized by frequent interruptions or a wide diversity of disassociated usage.

(13) Open End — Comments or remarks explaining a special situation.

**Table 6-2** Summary of Ranges, Means, and Standard Deviations of Work Characteristics in Percentage of Actual Time

| Characteristic | Range | Mean | Standard Deviation |
|---|---|---|---|
| Inside | 49.5-98.7 | 78.6 | 12.6 |
| Outside | 1.3-50.6 | 21.4 | 12.6 |
| | | | |
| Alone | 10.4-48.7 | 23.7 | 9.1 |
| Admin. Colleague | 0-63.2 | 9.7 | 12.5 |
| Admin. Subordinate | 5.9-47.9 | 22.7 | 8.9 |
| Board Member | 0-15.4 | 4.7 | 4.0 |
| Community Member | 0-21.0 | 4.5 | 4.8 |
| Medical Personnel | 0-13.7 | 6.8 | 4.5 |
| Patients | 0-11.6 | 1.9 | 2.8 |
| Other | 0-16.6 | 6.6 | 5.2 |
| | | | |
| Fragmentation | | | |
| Omissions | | | |
| Multiple Categories | | | |
| Approx. | | 20.0 | |
| | | | |
| Paperwork | 3.9-46.7 | 15.9 | 9.2 |
| Conversing | 37.9-77.8 | 60.6 | 10.0 |
| Observing | 0-7.4 | 2.2 | 2.4 |
| Thinking Alone | 0.13.6 | 3.3 | 3.3 |
| Fragmentation | | | |
| Omissions | | | |
| Multiple Categories | | | |
| Approx. | | 18.0 | |

*Source:* W.F. Rohrs, "How Time Flies," *Hospital and Health Services Administration,* Winter 1979, p. 28. Used by permission of publisher.

**Table 6-3**  Summary of Ranges, Means, and Standard Deviations of Work
Characteristics in Actual Recorded Hours

| Characteristics | Range | Mean | Standard Deviation |
|---|---|---|---|
| Weekly hours | 37.3-57.0 | 47.2 | 4.2 |
| Extra hours | 0-8.5 | 3.3 | 4.8 |
| Inside | 22.5-47.5 | 36.8 | 5.3 |
| Outside | .5-23.0 | 10.4 | 6.1 |
| Alone | 4.8-24.3 | 11.3 | 4.6 |
| Admin. Colleague | 0-28.8 | 4.5 | 5.7 |
| Admin. Subordinate | 2.5-22.8 | 10.8 | 4.3 |
| Board Member | 0-7.8 | 2.2 | 1.9 |
| Community Member | 0-10.8 | 2.2 | 2.4 |
| Medical Personnel | 0-6.5 | 3.2 | 2.1 |
| Patients | 0-5.0 | .9 | 1.2 |
| Others | 0-8.5 | 3.1 | 2.5 |
| Paperwork | 2.0-21.3 | 7.5 | 4.3 |
| Conversing | 17.3-36.8 | 28.6 | 5.3 |
| Observing | 0-3.3 | 1.0 | 1.1 |
| Thinking Alone | 0-6.0 | 1.6 | 1.5 |

Figures 6-1, 6-2, and 6-3 show actual mean percentages of reported time use, inside and outside of hospitals, alone and with other categories of people, and performing work characteristics.

A review of these charts points out the high percentages of time spent alone and with administrative subordinates, and the small percentage of time devoted to medical personnel, community members, board members, and patients. Conversing was a most dominant work characteristic, accounting for a mean of 61 percent of time, while relatively little time was used for thinking alone and observing.

A second and different reporting form was also furnished to the respondents in order to obtain individual opinions concerning an ideal or preferred allocation of time for the same work characteristics as shown on the form for recording actual time use. Some minor modifications were necessary to preclude ambiguities and overcome inherent difficulties. These findings are summarized in Figures 6-4, 6-5, and 6-6.

**Figure 6-1** Mean Percentages of Actual Time Spent Inside and Outside of Employing Hospitals

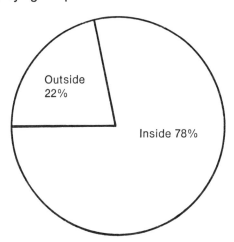

*Source:* W.F. Rohrs. "How Time Flies," *Hospital and Health Services Administration,* Winter 1979, p. 30. Used by permission of publisher.

---

**Figure 6-2** Mean Percentages of Actual Time Spent Alone and with Other Categories of People

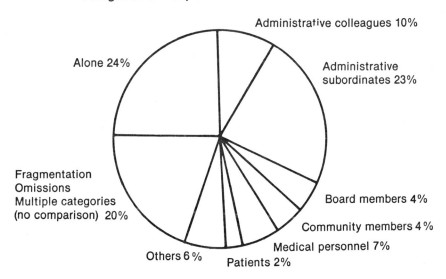

*Source:* W.F. Rohrs. "How Time Flies," *Hospital and Health Services Administration,* Winter 1979, p. 31. Used by permission of publisher.

**Figure 6-3** Mean Percentages of Actual Time Spent Performing Work
Characteristics

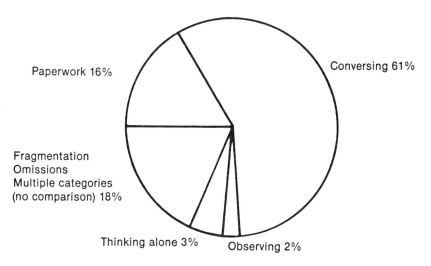

*Source:* W.F. Rohrs. "How Time Flies," *Hospital and Health Services Administration,*
Winter 1979, p. 33. Used by permission of publisher.

---

**Figure 6-4** Mean Percentages of Ideal Time Spent Inside and Outside of
Employing Hospitals

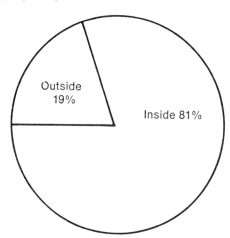

*Source:* W.F. Rohrs. "How Time Flies," *Hospital and Health Services Administration,*
Winter 1979, p. 30. Used by permission of publisher.

**Figure 6-5** Mean Percentages of Ideal Time Spent Alone and with Other Categories of People

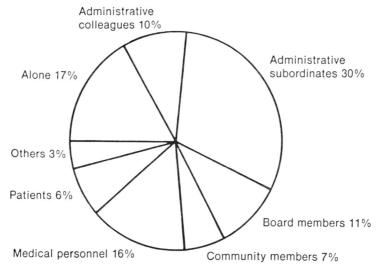

*Source:* W.F. Rohrs. "How Time Flies," *Hospital and Health Services Administration*, Winter 1979, p. 31. Used by permission of publisher.

**Figure 6-6** Mean Percentages of Ideal Time Spent Performing Work Characteristics

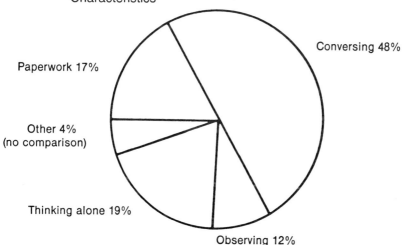

*Source:* W.F. Rohrs. "How Time Flies," *Hospital and Health Services Administration*, Winter 1979, p. 33. Used by permission of publisher.

Comparing the actual with the ideal mean percentages of time allocation does not reveal any great desire for major change in terms of where time was spent, i.e., inside or outside of the employing institutions. For the categories of alone and with other people, however, some changes seem desirable. Ideally, time spent alone and in fragmented periods should be reduced. Conversely, more time was desired for administrative subordinates, medical personnel, board members, community members, and patients. Finally, for work characteristics, conversing was seen as too high, with observing and thinking alone deserving of more time.

A more detailed analysis of the data indicates that no overall drastic adjustments to existing patterns of time use were advocated. But, because of isolated instances of individual administrators who recommended substantial changes, it is suggested comparisons between actual and ideally allocated time use be considered primarily on an individual basis.

Because this study of hospital administrators was based on a small convenience sample, the findings and implications pertain only to this group of volunteers, and are not therefore applicable to all hospital administrators in general, and should not be considered as such. No implications should be drawn from this study for overcoming the difficulty of evaluating a hospital administrator's performance on the basis of time utilization. Many variables beyond the scope of this investigation may be operative in one situation and perhaps be negligible in another. Evaluation of performance was not an objective of this research. No optimal use of time is either stated or should be inferred from the findings, as the research is purely descriptive.

## THE MINTZBERG STUDY

At this point, it may be helpful to contrast the previous data and implications with the recent work of Henry Mintzberg with regard to characteristics of managerial work (1980, p. 30).

> My own study of chief executives found no break in the pace of activity during office hours. The mail (average of 36 pieces per day), telephone calls (average of 5 per day), and meetings (average of 8) accounted for almost every minute from the moment these men entered their offices in the morning until they departed in the evenings. A true break seldom occurred. Coffee was taken during meetings, and lunchtime was almost always devoted to formal or informal meetings. When free time appeared, everpresent subordinates quickly usurped it.
>
> Thus the work of managing an organization may be described as taxing. The quantity of work to be done, or that the manager chooses to do, during the day is substantial and the pace is unrelenting.

Why do managers adopt this pace and workload? One major reason is the inherently openended nature of the job. The manager is responsible for the success of his organization, and there are really no tangible mileposts where he can stop and say, "Now my job is finished."

No matter what kind of managerial job he has, he always carries the nagging suspicion that he might be able to contribute just a little bit more. Hence he assumes an unrelenting pace in his work (Mintzberg, 1980, p. 30).

The brevity of many of the manager's activities is also most surprising. Figure 6-7 shows the distribution of activities by duration for the chief executives of our study. Half of the observed activities were completed in less than 9 minutes, and only one tenth took more than an hour. In effect, the managers were seldom able or willing to spend much time on any one issue in any one session. Telephone calls were brief and to the point (averaging 6 minutes), and desk work sessions and unscheduled meetings seldom lasted as long as half an hour (they averaged 15 and 12 minutes, respectively). Only scheduled meetings, usually dealing with a multitude of issues or one complex issue, commonly took more than an hour. But even an average duration of 68 minutes seems meager, given the nature of the issues discussed. The same characteristic of brevity was reflected in the treatment of mail. A few of the men expressed dislike for long memos, and most long reports and periodicals were skimmed quickly.

Managers also frequently interrupted their desk work to place telephone calls or to request that subordinates come by. One chief executive located his desk so that he could look down a long hallway. The door was usually open, and his subordinates were continually coming into his office. He fully realized that by moving this desk, closing his door, or changing the rules his secretary used to screen callers he could easily have eliminated many of these interruptions (Mintzberg, 1980, p. 34).

Why, then, is there indication that managers prefer brevity and interruption in their work? To some extent, certainly, the manager tolerates interruption because he does not wish to discourage the flow of current information. Furthermore, the manager may become accustomed to the variety in his work, and he may find that boredom develops easily. But it would appear that these factors can only partly explain the manager's behavior.

A more significant explanation might be that the manager becomes conditioned by his workload. He develops a sensitive appreciation for the opportunity cost of his own time—the benefits forgone by doing one thing instead of another. Thus, he takes on much work because he realizes his own worth to the organization. In addition, he is aware of the everpresent assortment of obligations associated with his job—the mail that cannot be delayed, the callers that must be attended to, the

**Figure 6-7** Frequency Distribution of Managerial Activities by Duration*

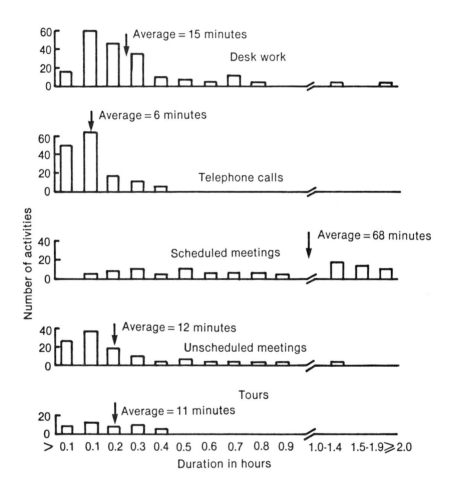

*Based on five weeks of observation of chief executives' work.

*Source:* H. Mintzberg, *The Nature of Managerial Work,* Prentice-Hall, Inc., 1980, p. 33. Used by permission of author.

meetings that require his participation. In other words, no matter what he is doing, the manager is plagued by what he might do and what he must do.

In effect, the manager is encouraged by the realities of his work to develop a particular personality—to overload himself with work, to do things abruptly, to avoid wasting time, to participate only when the value of participation is tangible, to avoid too great an involvement with any one issue. To be superficial is, no doubt, an occupational hazard of managerial work. In order to succeed, the manager must, presumably, become proficient at this superficiality (Mintzberg, 1980, p. 35).

Managers appeared to interact quite freely with many subordinates and were not reluctant to "hurdle" the hierarchy in a downward fashion for needed contacts. This appears to be a cardinal principle, to be maintained by expediency as the overriding factor. Managers also spend a small amount of time with their own managers, with verbal contact quite limited.

We may summarize by characterizing the manager's position as the neck of an hourglass. Information and requests flow to him from a wide variety of outside contacts. He sits between this network of contacts and his organization, sifting what is received from the outside and sending much of it into his organization. Other informational inputs and requests come from below, some to be used by him, others to be sent back to different parts of the organization or outside to the manager's contact (Mintzberg, 1980, p. 48).

Mintzberg (1980) identified eight managerial types and analyzed how they spent their time:

1. *The Contact Man.* Some managers spend much of their time outside their organizations, dealing with people who can help them by doing them favors, giving them sales orders, providing privileged information, and so on. In addition, this type of manager expends much effort developing his reputation and that of his organization by giving speeches or doing favors himself. These individuals also serve as liaisons or figureheads.
2. *The Political Manager.* Another type of manager also spends a good part of his time with outsiders, but for different purposes. He is caught in a complex managerial position where he is required to reconcile a great many diverse political forces acting on his organization. This manager must spend a good part of his time in formal activities, meeting regularly with directors or the boss, receiving and negotiating with pressure groups, and explaining the actions of his organization to special interest parties. These individuals also serve as spokespersons or negotiators (p. 127).
3. *The Entrepreneur.* A third type of manager spends a good part of his time seeking opportunities and implementing changes in his organization. These individuals are also negotiators.

4. *The Insider.* Many managers are concerned chiefly with the maintenance of smooth-running internal operations. They spend their time building up structure, developing and training their subordinates, and overseeing the operations they develop. These individuals are resource allocators.

5. *The Real-Time Manager.* The primary concern of this manager is also with the maintenance of internal operations, but his time scale and problems are different. We can use the term real-time manager to describe that person who operates primarily in the present, devoting his efforts to ensuring that the day-to-day work of his organization continues without interruption. These individuals are also disturbance handlers (p. 128).

6. *The Team Manager.* There is another type of manager who is oriented to the inside, but has a special concern. He is preoccupied with the creation of a team that will operate as a cohesive whole and will function effectively. These individuals assume the role of leader.

7. *The Expert Manager.* In some situations a manager must perform an expert role in addition to his regular managerial roles. As head of a specialist staff group this manager must serve as a center of specialized information in the larger organization. He advises other managers and is consulted on specialized problems. This individual also serves as a monitor and/or spokesman.

8. *The New Manager.* Our last type of manager is the one in a new job. Lacking contacts and information at the beginning, the ''new manager'' concentrates on the liaison and monitor roles in an attempt to build up a web of contacts and a data base. The decisional roles cannot become fully operative until he has more information. When he does, he is likely to stress the entrepreneur role for a time, as he attempts to put his distinct stamp on his organization. Then he may settle down to being one of the other managerial types—contact man, insider, or some other type (p. 129).

In recent years the job of a hospital administrator has become increasingly complex as more and more decision-making responsibilities have been added to an already burdensome workload. With the adoption and implementation of various skills and techniques borrowed from disciplines such as management, marketing, finance, and accounting, the image of the hospital administrator now more clearly mirrors that of a business executive who is involved in the operation of a profit-oriented enterprise.

One interesting way to view this resemblance is to compare the similarities and differences in how business managers and hospital administrators utilize their time. As a basis for this analysis, appropriate findings from various prior research projects, cited above, and the present study are presented in Figures 6-8 through 6-11.

Figure 6-8, which shows the total average number of weekly hours worked, indicates a high degree of uniformity. This is particularly interesting when it is

**Figure 6-8** Average Weekly Hours

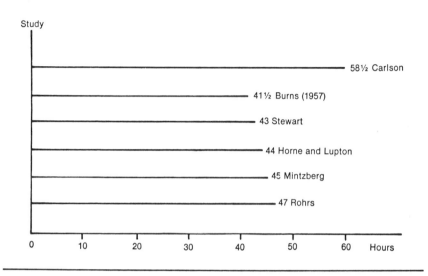

recalled that the various studies span more than two decades, and the data were generated from widely diversified sources.

Figure 6-9 displays a similar consistency in the average percentage of time spent inside the organization. Horne and Lupton have this comment about their respondents (1965, p. 28):

> A picture of an "organization man" homeward bound, with bulging briefcase, preparing to sacrifice his family life for the firm, is not suggested by the evidence. He may take a bulging briefcase home but he hardly ever opens it. Nor does he seem to be busy winning friends and influencing people for work purposes or special occasions outside the organization.

The average percentage working time spent alone is presented in Figure 6-10. As previously stated, the differences are not large. Stewart (1967, pp. 50-51) makes this statement about time spent alone:

> There are jobs that one would expect to involve a relatively large amount of time alone. These are the so-called, "backroomjobs" which require a high proportion of managerial work. . . . There are other jobs, such as that of general manager, whose holders are likely to spend little time alone.

**Figure 6-9**  Percentage of Working Time Spent Inside Own
Organization

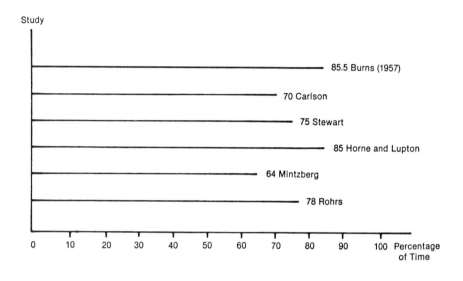

**Figure 6-10**  Percentage of Working Time Spent Alone

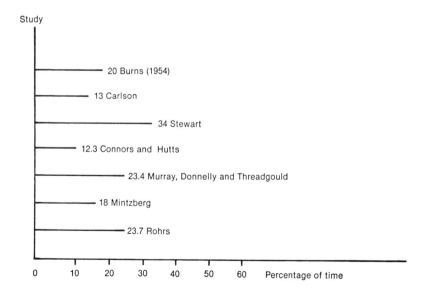

Time spent with subordinates is portrayed in Figure 6-11. A slightly wider range of percentages occurs in this category. In this connection, Carlson (1951, p. 54) notes the following about his Swedish executives:

> Conferences and private talks with visitors in the office were also the most time consuming of the various occupations recorded for all but three of the executives, and most of these visitors were subordinates.

Only a few earlier researchers gathered data which characterized the performance of work, and therefore except for paperwork and conversing, little information is available for comparative purposes. Figure 6-12 indicates the average percentage of time used for paperwork. Again, in this category, the variations are small. In commenting about paperwork, Stewart states (p. 38):

> A SEA OF PAPER? Yes for some, no for others. Managers varied enormously in the amount of time they spent on writing, dictating, reading and figurework.

**Figure 6-11** Percentage of Working Time Spent with Subordinates

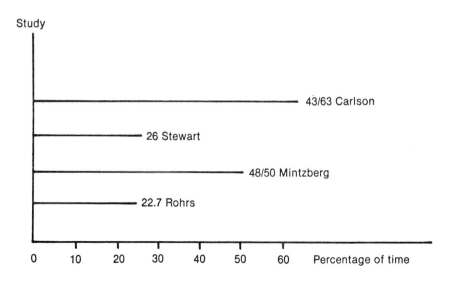

**Figure 6-12** Percentage of Working Time Spent Doing Paperwork

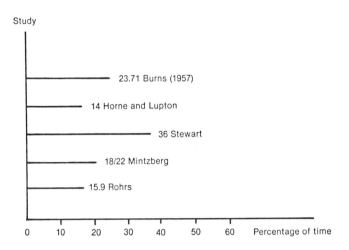

An interesting further observation by Horne and Lupton (pp. 25-26) concerning paperwork:

> The managers in general recorded themselves as having spent little time dealing with paper. . . . About one-fifth of their working time is spent reading. Since we have no information about what they read, this item is difficult to evaluate, but information . . . would suggest that it would be closely connected with getting things done—information about progress or lack of it, reports and the like.

Figure 6-13 compares data about the work characteristic conversing. All the studies shown indicate substantial agreement at a high level of time use.

A brief review of some overall comparisons will direct attention to interesting differences and similarities. The 24 hospital administrators in the Rohrs study, in general, averaged a longer work week than the individuals surveyed by most of the other researchers. These administrators spent about the same proportion of time inside their own organizations as reported by other studies and the percentage of time alone is quite consistent with prior findings. A close similarity also exists between the hospital administrators' time spent with subordinates when matched

**Figure 6-13** Percentage of Working Time Spent Conversing

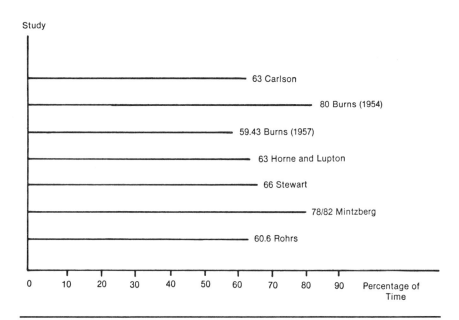

Study

```
0    10   20   30   40   50   60   70   80   90   Percentage of
                                                   Time
```

- 63 Carlson
- 80 Burns (1954)
- 59.43 Burns (1957)
- 63 Horne and Lupton
- 66 Stewart
- 78/82 Mintzberg
- 60.6 Rohrs

with Stewart's results, although overall some modest disparity with other research is evident. The percentage of time spent on paperwork and conversing, however, is relatively close to the findings of the other investigators.

An examination of comments entered on the time logs by the individual hospital administrators confirms observations of earlier researchers who described the fast and constant tempo of work, marred by frequent interruptions in the midst of a rapidly changing milieu, and demanding a wide diversity of interests, activities, skills, and time.

It is appropriate to end this chapter with Henry Mintzberg's conclusion (1973, p. 30):

> The work of managing an organization may be described as taxing. The quantity of work to be done, or that the manager chooses to do, during the day is substantial and the pace is unrelenting. After hours, the chief executive (and probably many other managers as well) appears to be able to escape neither from an environment that recognizes the power and status of his position nor from his own mind, which has been well trained to search continuously for new information.

Some suggestions of Mintzberg conclude this chapter on managerial roles by suggesting that managing, time effectiveness, and role clarification are key components of this complex process. The manager's time assumes an enormous opportunity cost. Lacking time, he can inhibit organizational development by postponing requests for authorization, by delaying improvement projects, by reducing the amount of information he disseminates, and so on. It appears, therefore, that management scientists can usefully turn their attention to the manager's scheduling activity. By bringing more consistency to the manager's schedule, by relieving him of much of the need to schedule his own work, and by using systematic analysis to design his schedule in accordance with his needs and those of this organization, the management scientist can achieve considerable gains in efficiency. In fact, it is surprising that there has been so little analytical effort in this area, considering the extent to which the activities of other works in the organization have been studied.

A scheduling program would involve (1) determining the manager's time constraints, (2) defining and categorizing the demands for his time, and (3) developing a set of adaptable scheduling rules to control time allocation. Step one can easily be achieved by having the manager specify such things as his working hours and his attitude toward evening and lunchtime work. Likewise, it would be a simple matter to categorize the various demands for a manager's time (Mintzberg, 1980, pp. 146-147).

---

**REFERENCES**

American Hospital Association. *The American Hospital Association guide to the health care field* (1975 Ed.). Chicago: The American Hospital Association, 1975.

Barnard, C.I. *The functions of the executive*. Cambridge, Mass.: Harvard University Press, 1978, 163; 128-129.

Burns, T. The directions of activity and communication in a departmental executive group. *Human Relations*, February 1954, *7*, 78.

Burns, T. Management in action. *Operational Research Quarterly*, June 1957, *8*, 48, 60.

Carlson, S. *Executive behavior*. Stockholm: C.A. Stronberg Aktiebolag, 1951.

Copeman, G., Luijk, H., & Hanika, F. de P. *How the executive spends his time*. London: Business Publications Ltd., 1963.

Dolson, M.T. How hospital administrators rate different tasks. *Modern Hospital*, June 1965, 96.

Drucker, P.F. *The effective executive*. New York: Harper and Row, 1967, 35.

Forrest, C.R., Johnson, A.C., & Mosher, J. The changing role of the hospital administrator. *Proceedings of the 36th Annual Meeting of Academy of Management*, 1976, 435.

Gulick, L.H. Notes on the theory of organization. In L.H. Gulick & L.F. Urwick (Eds.), *Papers on the science of administration*. New York: Columbia University Press, 1973.

Horne, J.H., & Lupton, T. The work activities of middle managers—An exploratory study. *The Journal of Management Studies*, February 1965, *2*, 25, 26, 28.

Mintzberg, H. *The nature of managerial work*. New York: Harper and Row, 1973.

Mintzberg, H. *The nature of managerial work*. Englewood Cliffs, N.J.: Prentice-Hall, 1980.

Murray, R.T., Donnelly, P.R., and Threadgould, M. How administrators spend their time. *Hospital Progress*, September 1968, 49.

Rohrs, W.F. How time flies. *Hospital and Health Services Administration*, Winter 1979, 28, 30, 31, 33.

Stewart, R. *Managers and their jobs*. London: Macmillan and Co., 1967.

Taylor, F.W. *The principles of scientific management*. New York: W.W. Norton and Co., 1911.

Toward a more effective management. United Hospital Fund of New York, 1973.

Yanda, R.L. *Doctors as managers of health teams*. New York: AMACOM, 1977, 29, 119, 122.

# Chapter 7

# Managing Health Care Objectives

TIME MANAGEMENT HIGHLIGHTS

1. Management by Objectives (MBO) is a process intended to bring about formulation of clear goals, development of realistic action plans to achieve goals, and the necessary steps to actualize results. It is closely linked to participative management and develops a commitment to the organization.

2. It is crucial to balance a variety of needs and goals in every area where performance and results directly and vitally affect the survival and prosperity of the organization. These objectives must be defined in terms of the manager's contribution to the overall unit of which he is a part.

3. The process of formulating objectives is a matter of asking yourself the right question, or at least, not asking the wrong question. Good objectives are measured by time, innovation, quantity, and quality.

4. The medical care administrator must specify his objectives, choose appropriate ones, resolve conflict among objectives, and keep them operational and current to adapt to changing needs. These health care objectives are often vaguely defined, complex, in constant flux, and internally inconsistent—all affecting time.

5. Managers do not plan for the setting of objectives because they are often extremely orthodox and rigid in their thinking, which makes it difficult for them to make organizational decisions. Managers who have not been socialized by the traditional methods of managing appear to do much better in MBO programs.

6. MBO is a systems approach to managing an organization. It is not a technique and goes far beyond mere budgeting. The objectives are states of individual motivation derived from the needs of a par-

ticular individual. The objectives are values to be achieved by the individual and organization as well.

7. The output of an employee of a health care organization is difficult to determine and becomes problematic when objectives are to be stated. Before pay can be related to production, a viable method of measuring individual performance must be utilized.

8. Group goal setting may be essential since the goals of a health care organization personify the image of a well-managed institution. Goals should be defined as to the amount and direction of change that is desired in a given period of time. This is a needs analysis.

9. When MBO is used properly, the manager of a department is not needed on a daily basis to make things happen since the conceptual blueprint has been clearly outlined. If a health care manager is needed for every major decision, then the institution is ineffective and time is being wasted.

10. Goals and objectives must be specific; defined in terms of measurable results; linked to overall organization goals; have a specific time period for review and accomplishment; be flexible; have a plan of action to accomplish results; and be prioritized.

11. Goals within hospitals need to be:
    a. balanced and extensive
    b. directed toward measurement
    c. present and future oriented
    d. designed for guidance
    e. in touch with the environment
    f. based upon consensus
    g. in keeping with the principle of disclosure
    h. focused upon results
    i. subject to continuous monitoring

12. As long as managers only appraise the end result of an operation, without giving adequate weight to the means, there will be problems with this process.

13. A new appraisal system may be needed which is based on behavioral job descriptions in place of the traditional substantive method which has created problems and dysfunction.

14. The MBO interview process is crucial for the legitimization of this process, where objectives can be negotiated in a reality-based manner and even openly renegotiated. This commitment is also essential for the feedback element of this process. Without feedback, support and control are virtually diluted within this effort.

15. The guidelines for actually developing an MBO must include the quantitative statement of an attainable objective with an

accompanying weight for priority. Also, standards of performance and terminal dates are suggested for solidifying the agreement between the parties.

One of the efficient and effective methods of increasing managerial expertise and skill is by the adoption of a managerial and behavioral process commonly referred to as management by objectives. This process, when executed in the most professional manner by skilled health care managers, is an important component in developing a model intended to reduce ambiguity, anxiety, and the wasting of time. While management by objectives (commonly referred to as MBO) has its roots in the industrial domain, its application to government agencies and health care institutions is now quite common and studies will be presented indicating some success in this utilization. While focusing on MBO in the health care domain, however, we will also draw from the organizational model that has proven to be valid and reliable.

Recent research has highlighted the fact that there is a direct relationship between the clarity of organizational goals and business success. High-growth organizations develop clear objectives and undertake to accomplish them. Gordon and Goldberg (1977, p. 41) found that organizational clarity—clear goals, formal planning, complete planning, and existence of defined plans—leads to high performance. Due to the fact that human beings are not always logical, the process of formulating objectives seldom follows a set plan. Basically, formulating objectives is a matter of asking yourself the right question, or at least not asking the wrong question. The most difficult problems in management arise not from failures of problem analysis but from failures arising from solving the wrong problem (Kelly, 1980, p. 101). MBO is widely used not only in the United States but in Canada, Britain, Europe, and Japan. Its appeal is based largely on its common-sense approach and its simplistic format. It is valuable because it enables planning to take place at a fairly low level in the organization, provides a valid review of progress, improves motivation and commitment, focuses organizations on the achievement of results, increases interaction between managers and their subordinates, and, last but not least, creates a pleasant and stimulating climate (Kelly, p. 113). This endorsement connotes effectiveness, efficiency, and a productive environment where time is a valuable resource and not wasted due to fragmented directives and goals which are suboptimized (Appelbaum, 1975, p. 13). Suboptimization occurs when group goals assume priority over organizational goals. Resulting conflict occurs when objectives are nebulous and competition between groups is encouraged.

The medical care administrator has certain responsibilities with regard to the objectives of his program. These include (1) specification of objectives, (2) the choice of objectives, (3) resolution of conflict among objectives, (4) rendering objectives operational, and (5) keeping them current by adaptation to changing needs and conditions. This does not mean that all these responsibilities rest on the administrator alone, but that he is a major participant in discharging them (Donabedian, 1973, p. 43).

Although the health care manager may have a number of strategies to choose from, he has a single aim: to measure and evaluate performance in terms of results, not effort. The manager does this by creating an output process that embraces:

- setting performance standards

- establishing systems of measurement

- acquiring sufficient operational information (not merely data)

- maintaining consistency in evaluating outcomes

- bringing the concept of feedback control into play

- taking corrective action and following through on changes introduced

The results expected and methods of evaluating results are considered here with the output of the system and its relationship to purposes. It is important that objectives be results oriented and measurable in nature, where possible (Bennett, 1978, p. 145).

This is an essential operation for health care managers since hospitals deal with people, with lives, and with patient care. The goal is not increased production, increased sales, or increased profits. But before one can correctly conclude that the methods of General Motors or other business managers cannot be helpful, one must first demonstrate that industry does not also deal with people; with lives; and with the physical, emotional, and ecological well-being of people (Deegan, 1977, p. 2). The environment of a hospital is quite complex, based upon the interrelated services and value systems of those working within it. The complexities and dynamics of this environment create a system of management that is intended to focus more on results and less on activities. The essence of this is a management by objectives orientation.

MBO is not a new fad or concept. In fact it is based upon a logical, common-sense philosophy and most competent managers do apply its principles, even if they do not refer to it as MBO. However, many managers work toward their own departmental objectives rather than toward the overall company objectives, which often creates a disparity between the two. Also, many people never know what objectives they are trying to achieve, and this is counterproductive, time-consuming, and costly.

The term MBO was first used by Peter Drucker in *The Practice of Management* in 1954. He introduced three major points in this book relating to the approach:

1. For a business to be successful, all managers' jobs must be directed towards the objectives of the business.
2. Managers should set their own objectives and be able to control their own future.
3. Management development is essentially self-development of the manager under the guidance of the boss.

Not until the mid-1960s did systems develop that could incorporate Drucker's ideas effectively.

At the very outset the administrator is faced with the problem of distinguishing objectives from the means used to attain them. Simon (1961, pp. 62-66) has pointed out that the problem arises from the partially ordered nature of the underlying phenomenon. There is, according to this formulation, a hierarchy of events such that each item in a chain is partly or wholly dependent on the one that precedes it and contributes, in varying degrees, to the one that follows. The distinction between means and ends is thus effaced, so that each level in a chain can be viewed either as a means or as an end, depending on which is more relevant to the purposes at hand.

Health care administrators must recognize that the objectives of an organization (or objectives within an organization) are indeed complex, vaguely defined, in constant flux, and often internally inconsistent. It is also recognized that objectives formulated at one level in an organization may be modified at another level and further modified, even subverted, in actual execution. The diversity of goals has to be recognized (Donabedian, 1973, p. 32). There is another problem in the anlysis of organizational goals resulting from the discrepancy between the official goals of the health care organization and the operative or real goals.

The tendency for organizations to deviate from their legitimate and avowed purposes is a general tendency referred to as "goal displacement." The inference is that the legitimate and avowed purposes are thereby less well served. A frequent form of goal displacement is when concern for the survival and welfare of the organization itself takes precedence over the broader objectives which the organization ostensibly exists to serve. Another is undue emphasis on procedures as if they were ends in themselves rather than means to a larger service objective. Procedures may also be subverted to serve unintended goals (Donabedian, 1973, p. 35). A study was conducted (Scheff, 1962, pp. 208-217) which describes how, in a mental hospital, staff-patient conferences and tranquilizing drugs were used to control patients rather than to further their rehabilitation as originally intended by the professional staff.

This situation brings about the need for hospitals to establish satisfactory management concepts and techniques related to a determination of where they want to go and how they get there. This is so great that the failure of health care executives to exhibit adequate development of these techniques is somewhat surprising. Many hospitals sustain serious organizational inadequacies and prolong the absence of acquiring the means to establish goals and achieve objectives. To go on without setting goals, without planning, without setting priorities, without measuring outcomes must be viewed as symptoms of mismanagement, particularly in the face of the continuing problems embedded in the organizational processes of communication, coordination, and control (Bennett, 1978, p. 79).

The frustrations, and very often the failures, experienced by adminstrators have stemmed from misdirection and misunderstanding of the purposes, meaning, and import of the body of principles embraced by the concept of management by objectives. Specifically:

> What needs to be understood . . . is that managing with goals and objectives is a concept that is philosophical, not mechanical, in nature. It is a process (not a program) based on commitment, rather than compliance. It is an approach that is evolutionary, not instant; motivational, not restraining; and integral, not independent (Bennett, 1976, p. 67).

The process of setting objectives is important in helping the manager within the health care environment to differentiate between what should be and what is. This system of personal responsibility is essential since results are the measure utilized in allocating the rewards and human resources of the hospital. These results are often used for the approving of new programs, modifying some programs, or eliminating programs that have proven to be unfeasible or unworkable. Overall organizational objectives, once they are developed and applied, are crucial elements in the success of a health care organization. They provide the foundation for selecting and allocating of resources and they also serve as foundations for long- and short-range goals, policies, and procedures. These plans are often used to help the organization evaluate the performance and progress of those resources. These activities assist the management of a health care institution in guiding operations and planning for future contingencies. Therefore, it is important that precise objectives and subgoals are agreed upon by the parties involved, or individual efforts may not contribute to the essential overall success of the organization. These broad-based goals must be translated into specific, achievable objectives that are realistic and that can be actualized.

Objectives serve as the basis for solidarity and stability. The integrative function of certain shared objectives ensures stability. Agreement over objectives unites the activities of individuals and groups within an organization. Disagreement over objectives, or inconsistency and conflict among objectives, results in stress, conflict, and instability. A study of entrepreneurial medical groups focused upon this issue (Du Bois, 1967, pp. 8-9).

Successful groups were found to have had clearly formulated objectives. These objectives were expressed to recruits in the recruitment process and tended to help in the selection of recruits willing to serve the stated organizational objectives. In the establishment of group policies and the resolution of management problems, organizational objectives served as a basis for judgment. The nature of the objectives served by the highly viable medical groups was distinctly professional. Financial success for physician participants, leisure, professional advancement and relative status all were important aspirations implicit in the group structure, but professional excellence, patient service, the practice of "good" medicine, were the principal objectives and the ultimate criteria for decision making. . . . Diminished viability or non-viability can result from organizational objectives which lead to organizational policies in conflict with the professional role or from failure to define or support organizational objectives as a central theme around which the organization is operated.

The process of MBO appears on the surface to be simplistic, but the dynamic impact of the internal environment and other intraorganizational interactions leads to certain problems. The nature of management involves coordinating the activities of individuals toward the attainment of objectives and goals. The manager has, as his major task, the definition and interpretation of broad organizational goals and the translation of these into operational goals for his subordinates. The necessary integration of these objectives must be completely understood by everyone involved and must have the commitment of top management. If not, there occurs confusion, dysfunctional behavior, aborted missions, and the wasting of time.

## MBO: TECHNIQUE AND THEORY

Management by objectives is actually a philosophy of management developed by multiple theories and proven techniques. It is not a reactive way of managing an organization, since this approach is costly, risky, and time-consuming. The emphasis on MBO is the attempt to predict and influence the contingencies that affect the organization rather than react to events that have already occurred. A major focus should be directed toward change and improving the organizational and individual contributions of this system. The MBO process is important for a participative management system since it is an interdependent and interrelated system based upon (1) the formulation of clear statements of objectives, (2) the development of realistic action plans needed to achieve these objectives, (3) the systematic management and measurement of achievement and performance, and (4) the taking of necessary steps to actualize the results.

MBO is closely related to participative management as a theory and technique intended to give employees adequate input about problems affecting their careers and welfare and to improve the organizational climate more effectively. A feeling of personal significance, involvement, and having an input into the overall operation can lead individuals to develop not only a sense of commitment to the organization, but also a desire to see it achieve. Feelings of pride in one's organization are not overly common in health care organizations, but participative efforts can help illuminate those feelings. These positive attitudes tend to prevent or reverse the frequently negative effects of unresolved conflict battles.

Some specific advantages include:

- improved morale

- more efficient communication up and down the organization

- earlier detection and action on operational problems

- simultaneous improvement in worker satisfaction and productivity

- increased trust between employees and managers

- reduced absenteeism and turnover

- greater willingness on the part of management to institute changes beneficial to workers

- greater employee support of management plans and actions

- improvement in the competitive position of a company through greater operating efficiency

- making the MBO program alive and legitimate via participation

The MBO process is a system of management intended to illuminate planning, controlling, organizing, problem solving, decision making, and motivation. It is a system that allows certain aspects of organizational processing to be handled in a logical, systematic, and human manner which helps maintain efficiency. Management by and with objectives is also an extremely important aspect of controlling organizational processes and its costs. While health care administrators who are not medically trained often assume the role of the administrator in a hospital, it is the physician who has managed the health care organization and has made key operating decisions, even though he seems inappropriately trained for this role. The following is an account of a consultant working within a health care institution who worked with medical staff on managerial processes (Herzlinger, 1978, p. 107).

In the past years we have taught accounting and finance to hundreds of doctors who have charge of large and powerful healthcare institutions. Although they are enormously talented and industrious individuals, very few could read or understand his or her own financial statements. The sums wasted because of lack of managerial skills must be substantial. Conversely, the acquisition of general management skills by doctors will enormously enhance the efficiency and effectiveness of the health-care system. Training and organizational behavior, financial mechanisms, investment management, and techniques for capital and operating budgeting are easy to acquire.

This process actually links together many aspects of management tasks and responsibilities which usually fall under the control of the health care administrator. In a recent statement Peter Drucker, considered to be one of the architects of Management by Objectives, stated his feeling that the solution to the problem of the hospital lies in thinking through objectives and priorities (Drucker, 1977, p. 140). Drucker appears to suggest that the job of management is to balance a variety of needs and goals in every area where performance and results directly and vitally affect the survival and prosperity of the organization.

The first prerequisite to managing is determining what you want to accomplish through your management unit or, in other words, the actual objectives for the unit. Drucker's contention was that these objectives should be defined in terms of the manager's contribution to the overall unit of which he is a part. Therefore, to assure that unit goals are congruent with the total organization, each manager must develop objectives supporting the objectives of the next higher unit, or as Rensis Likert (1967) hypothesized, develop a linking process. Drucker further evaluated MBO in his classic work *The Practice of Management* (1954) and described the total process as follows (pp. 128-129): The goal of each manager's job must be defined by the contribution he has to make to the success of the larger unit of which he is a part. This requires each manager to develop and set the objectives of his unit himself. Higher management must of course reserve the power to approve or disapprove these objectives. But their development is part of a manager's responsibility; indeed, it is his first responsibility. It means too that every manager should responsibly participate in the development of the objectives of the higher unit of which he also is a part. Precisely because his aim should reflect the objective needs of the business, rather than merely what the individual manager wants, he must commit himself to them with a positive act of assent. He must know and understand the ultimate organizational goals, what is expected of him and why, what he will be measured against and how. This can be achieved when each of the contributing managers is expected to think through what the unit objectives are and is led, in other words, to participate actively and responsibly in the work of defining them. Only if his lower managers participate in this way can the higher manager know what to expect of them and make exacting demands.

This concern with top management commitment to, and participation in, MBO is essential. Top management's overriding responsibility for overall organizational planning has long been recognized by management theorists and practitioners alike.

In an excellent and comprehensive treatment of MBO, Dr. George Steiner made the following observations (Raia, 1974, p. 29):

1. Corporate planning will fail in the absence of the chief executive's support, participation, and guidance.
2. Corporate planning is the responsibility of the chief executive and cannot be delegated to a planning staff.
3. The chief executive is responsible for assuring that a proper organization for planning is created, that the manner of its functioning is clear and understood, and that it operates efficiently and effectively.
4. A chief executive must see that all managers understand that planning is a continuous function and not one pursued on an ad hoc basis or only during a formal planning cycle.
5. The chief executive should see that all managers recognize that planning means change, and the interaction of plans on people and institutions must be understood and considered.
6. Once plans are prepared, top management must make decisions on the basis of plans.

It is crucial that the chief executive officer in the health care organization provide the direction and impetus for an MBO program and commitment. Managers must become actively and supportively involved in formulating long-range goals (and even short-range goals) and strategic plans and in developing the mechanism for their implementation. This is essential to an MBO process that is based on an integrated system. As Drucker implied, these goals and the ensuing action help communicate to all members of the organization the level and intensity of the top management philosophy and commitment to the process of managing by objectives.

One of the most significant methods for implementing MBO is to know the basic foundation upon which it is built. Without the fundamental trust in employees that MBO requires, attempts to implement the system will be exercises in futility. Another important component is to understand how the total process functions. This process of implementation is based upon the basic assumption that the manager and his subordinate can reach agreement as to what must be accomplished. This notion also assumes that most people enjoy knowing what they are being held accountable for in achieving goals and do not enjoy investing time and effort on nebulous or inappropriate tasks. When top management defines and communicates the overall goals and objectives of the organization, the low-level managers should be able to develop appropriate objectives for the purpose of coordinating their unit's activities with overall organizational expectations (Ford & Bell, 1977, p. 16). Based upon this process, it is possible to ascertain the degree to which the objectives that an organization has set for itself have been achieved. Organizational effectiveness is actually the degree to which the organization, through its own efforts, realizes its objectives as specified by itself (Deniston et al., 1968, pp. 323-335). Also, for purposes of program evaluation, a clear distinction should be made between activities and objectives. Objectives require results-oriented behavior, while random activities are inefficient and waste time.

When objectives are not clarified, there is little linkage between effort and performance. Locke's research (1975) emphasizes the significance of establishing clear work goals. When the goals are not clear, administrative problems with attrition and resulting costs ensue. Dissatisfaction with the work itself, pay, promotion, and particularly lack of supervisory consideration are among the variables that stimulate thinking of quitting and intention to quit, the latter being the best predictor of actual attrition (Hollingsworth & Mobley, 1978, p. 348). When personnel begin to think about quitting, it affects their contributions, productivity, and time resourcefulness.

Given certain conditions, a strong and visible pay-performance link should be established. One of these conditions is the ability to operationalize performance. If a sound goal-setting process is utilized, the measurement of performance is facilitated. This in turn permits establishing a stronger pay-performance link (Hollingsworth & Mobley, p. 349). This point is essential as a component of increased productivity. Effective planning, widespread use of goal setting (MBO), and pay for performance are components of increasing productivity.

There are three steps to the process of formally establishing individual goals by all management personnel:

1. Agree on the objectives.
2. Put the goal down on paper.
3. Support a periodic review.

This MBO system impacts upon productivity and performance in the following ways:

- Forces consideration of good and bad performance in the most meaningful terms possible.

- Motivates the better employees through reinforcement for high performance.

- Identifies low performers so corrective action can be taken.

- Requires supervisors to manage their people fairly and deal with them openly in matters regarding pay and performance.

- Controls costs, acting to ensure that compensation dollars are paid for actual results produced (Conley & Miller, 1973, pp. 4-25).

- Ensures that hospital employees have clear work goals.

- Establishes link between pay increases and performance (primarily goal attainment).

- Equips managers to give performance feedback. The use of principles of reinforcement theory as they apply to supervisory performance feedback should be explored (Hollingsworth & Mobley, 1978, p. 350).

The MBO system and process, while being an effective tool for the health care administrator, can lead to some areas of conflict. The identification and resolution of conflict in objectives, as in other areas, is an everpresent task for the health care administrator. Fortunately for him, organizations appear to be able to tolerate a considerable degree of diversity in goals because (1) unifying objectives tend to be vague and ambiguous; (2) some objectives are stated in "nonoperational forms" that are "consistent with virtually any set of objectives" (Donabedian, 1973, p. 53); (3) there is compartmentalization, by function or otherwise, within the organization; (4) only a small set of goals is at issue at any given time, so that conflicting objectives do not often present themselves simultaneously; and (5) participants in a cooperative endeavor ("coalition") are willing to exchange some degree of attainment in some objectives to a higher degree of attainment in others. The place that ambiguity and lack of simultaneity occupy in this approach suggests that the explicit specification of objectives may exacerbate conflict. It is hoped, however, that in most instances such specification (at least by the administrator for himself) will lead to avoidance of conflict or its satisfactory resolution or containment (Donabedian, 1973, p. 53).

## RATIONAL PLANNING—A DIRECTION

MBO actually forces managers to communicate their needs and target goals to respective subordinates. The development and legitimization of objectives, however, is not a very creative process. Managers are considered to be functioning most effectively when they establish the goals that have to be reached and at the same time plot the path for the subordinate to reach these objectives. This usually results in a positive experience for both parties. The "path-goal theory of leadership" developed by Robert J. House and Terence R. Mitchell describes how a leader's behavior can have a motivating or satisfying impact on a subordinate's perception of his goals and the paths to those goals. A leader, through the use of positive and negative tasks and interpersonal rewards, can have a major impact on these perceptions. The leader can specify goals that are more or *less* attractive to a subordinate and can make it easy or difficult to attain these goals. Thus a leader can influence the type of outcomes experienced by the subordinate as well as clarifying the behavior-outcome relationship (Mitchell, 1978, p. 318). This process assists the manager of the organization in achieving some of the intricate elements of the job and the planning cycle. Managers have a tendency to perform programmed work at the expense of spontaneous work, and a good MBO system can add needed flexibility through the utilization of the contingency approach.

One of the problems encountered in MBO is that managers feel that once the planning has been achieved they can go back to their own work without any follow up. This connotes that planning is actually a separate process from doing. If this is the case then planning is such a unique and separate process that it cannot be integrated in the general workflow, which then allows this aspect of managing by objectives to become overlooked. When MBO is used in an organization successfully, the manager of a department is certainly not needed on a daily basis to make things happen since the conceptual blueprint has been clearly outlined. Indeed, if the health care manager is needed for every major decision, then the organization is ineffective and time is being wasted. MBO is an invaluable process when utilized in a health care environment because of its ability to reduce problems, and the general purpose of the manager is to achieve results in dealing with the identification of these problems. But the system does not work properly when the planning phase of MBO is not put into operation. Managers who do not plan for the setting of objectives often fail to do so because they quite incorrectly think that the process forces them to make a decision. In addition, they state that they do not have a basic philosophy about management and have not developed an effective managerial system. They are often extremely orthodox and rigid in their thinking, which makes it increasingly difficult for them to make organizational decisions.

Good objectives are measured by time, by innovation, and by quantity and quality of actualized decisions. Some objectives are based on individual motivation toward personal needs and values and are attached to individuals and not to organizations. Other objectives embody values that are defined by a major department or organization and constitute organizational objectives. MBO is an attempt to integrate these objectives and measure an individual's job effectiveness in relation to the overall goals of the organization.

In his book *How to Manage by Results* (1965), Dale McConkey states: "MBO is a systems approach to managing an organization—any organization." It is not a technique, or just another program, or a narrow area within the process of management. The MBO program must be an integrated, well-designed program that will be accepted by the managers of the organization for that very fact. For this to occur in a successful manner, the managers of the organization must have a personal investment in the MBO process. They must know what it is all about, what it is used for, and how it is interrelated with other organizational processes and functions such as performance evaluation, budgeting, salary administration, motivation, promotional review, and organizational effectiveness. The goals that are endorsed by top management are not always perceived by subordinate managers as possessing the same information or value systems. While most chief administrators are particularly interested in problem solving because they feel this is what they are being paid for, middle-level managers are more concerned with problem identification, which is the initial step in solving key problems. This duality is essential in the orientation and acceptance of the MBO program organizationally. Once the manager understands these key elements of the MBO process, he is taking the initial step in accepting and beginning to utilize it. This commitment leads to anticipated positive results through the mechanism of goal setting. With this as a direction, the emphasis is now future oriented and changing the organization becomes a major concern as well. Since an objective is a state or condition to be attained at some time in the future, more emphasis is placed on where the health care organization is going and also upon how it must reach this target through goal achievement.

Objectives should be thought of as clear statements of purpose and direction which are then formalized into a system of management. The goals may be either long or short range. They may be general, to provide direction to an entire organization, or they may be highly specific, to provide detailed direction for a given subordinate (Carroll & Tosi, 1973, p. 69). Managers in organizations generally set objectives for several reasons:

1. The clearer the direction of where you are trying to go, the greater the chance that you will get there. Also, progress can only be measured in terms of what you are attempting to achieve. The goals for the organization are the most difficult to establish. These goals must be based on future projections and a clear understanding regarding the organization's strengths and weaknesses. To do this, the organization must consider its economic forecast and outlook, which also includes an examination of the particular industry of which it is a part.

2. The human resources and financial constraints should be considered as well, since opportunities and problems that the organization may encounter will affect these elements in the future. This leads the manager to consider development of a program that will take advantage of future opportunities and at the same time handle present problems via a contingency approach. This total direction in planning could take the basic program and resources needed in the direction of the original plans.

3. A mechanism should be developed to revise the program and determine what secondary and tertiary objectives are needed for the organization in the future. At the time of a top management commitment, the plans must be transmitted to all levels of the organization. Before the manager can begin to enumerate measurable goals and objectives, he must be clear with regard to his ultimate purpose. In the health care setting, this means reviewing and restating the charter of the institution. It is the responsibility of the health care manager and his administrative team to be certain that the mission is well understood by all the managers and that all of the goals have been worked out with regard to the institutional purpose.

The health care administrator actually delegates the implementation of most responsibilities to various managers down the line. They will look at the "menu" or "charter" of hospital goals and use them as a point of reference in setting their own initial goals. The purpose of broad health care goals is to provide a stimulus to managers within the organization as to the responses and results expected from them. This often necessitates the setting of a priority listing so that everyone understands what is expected of them, thus reducing role conflict, ambiguity, and wasted time.

Health care administrators have often been asked what they perceive the basic goals or objectives of the hospital to be. Some cannot respond to this inquiry! It is essential that they perceive the quality of patient care and the efficient utilization of financial resources as primary objectives. General turnover rates for hospitals ranged from 36 to 72 percent approximately ten years ago, which was responsible for inefficient operations and spiralling costs. The need to reduce this variable is essential for health care managers and, therefore, turnover reduction today may be a logical objective in light of the efficient utilization of financial resources as a broad-based goal. The output of a health care employee is difficult to determine, which becomes problematic when objectives are to be stated. Output often becomes confused through the use of macro-type measures, and it is often erroneously measured by the amount of cost reduction attained over a period of time per employee. However, before pay can be related to productivity, a viable method of measuring individual performance must be utilized (Hand & Hollingsworth, 1978, p. 209).

## RESEARCH: MBO STUDIES

MBO attempts to link the functions of the health care manager and the overall mission of the organization. The development of an effective managerial climate is dependent upon the clarification of objectives to be achieved and a blueprint describing a route of how to get there. It seems reasonable to conclude that objective-oriented programs increase the clarity of job requirements, resulting in a greater satisfaction on the part of subordinates regarding the type of criteria to be used in their own evaluation. This event increases performance, efficiency, and the managing of resources in general.

This position was supported by several research studies attempting to demonstrate linkages between the setting of objectives and resulting conflict reduction within organizations.

## Study A

A study in human motivation and performance which has application in industry was conducted by Locke and Bryan (1967, pp. 120-130). They found that people responded better to specific goals rather than to abstract ones such as "do your best." Setting goals was found to be a possible antidote to boredom and a means of increasing motivation if manipulated properly. This laboratory study suggested that the best procedure is to use previous self-achievement of the worker as the base goal and to then encourage him to beat this previous level of performance. This prevents the frustration of attempting an impossible goal—which could be the result of random selection—yet it is high enough to stimulate interest and desire. In the end, such a procedure leads to higher output and higher satisfaction.

## Study B

Latham and Yukl (1975, pp. 824-845) completed an empirical study on goal setting and reviewed 27 articles providing strong support for Locke's propositions that specific goals increase performance and that difficult goals result in better performance than do easy goals. The studies did not provide evidence for Locke's proposition that goal setting mediates the effects of participation, monetary incentives, and performance feedback. However, there is some evidence that goal setting and feedback affect learning and motivation. The research indicated that goal-setting procedures are effective over an extended time period in a variety of organizations. Reward contingencies were important, as was participative goal setting in several studies. Goal setting can be difficult in highly complex jobs where accurate performance measures are not readily available. Consequently, goal setting with managers has been less successful than with nonmanagerial employees.

Management support, the interrelationships among jobs in the organization, and individual traits of the employee are all limiting conditions that may moderate the success of a goal-setting program as evidenced by this research survey.

## Study C

An in-depth survey (Kiev, 1974) of 150 executives drawn from organizations on *Fortune*'s list of major corporations explored a number of stress-related factors, including: psychological stress, self-defeating behavior, corporate limitations and objectives, the management of personnel, mechanisms for change, firing and retirement, and the corporation versus the individual. Study conclusions included the following:

- Corporate and personal goals should not be confused.
- Self-actualization through worthwhile performance is the best motivational strategy.
- Rules and temperaments should blend.
- Conflict is usually neither useful nor productive.
- An individual should be encouraged to assume responsibilities commensurate with his ability.

## Study D

A number of studies conducted in hospitals and industry have illustrated the importance of job satisfaction to turnover. A study at the Mount Sinai Hospital in New York City (Hand & Hollingsworth, 1978, p. 212) found four major causes of employee separation: unsatisfactory interpersonal relationships, dissatisfaction with ratings, dissatisfaction with pay systems, and general disappointment related to expectations. There appears to be a direct link between developing job performance measures based upon goals and individual levels of satisfaction and/or dissatisfaction.

## Study E

Other research (Meglino, 1977, pp. 22-28) was conducted highlighting goals, performance, and several common managerial concepts in light of recent information concerning the effects of stress and performance. The perceived level of stress is subjective, depending on the individual appraisals of employees. Thus, simple statements regarding the impact of rewards on performance are not always true. Major attention should be given to evaluation methods. Managers should try to maintain low levels of stress for employees who have not had sufficient time to learn their jobs well, and for those with very difficult tasks. When excessive stress is obvious, the manager may take the following steps to help to alleviate it:

- Adjust standards for quantity or quality.

- Reduce job responsibility.

- Separate the review process from normal contact with the employee.

- Clarify performance standards as much as possible via objective setting.

It is clear from this research that goal setting is an extremely important process in the total MBO experience. The goals of the health care organization illuminate and project the image of a well-managed institution.

## SELF-APPRAISAL

To check the completeness of the setting of goals, department heads and middle managers in the health care institution may examine the following issues by considering some provoking questions:

- If I were the executive director of the hospital, which key result areas in my own department would I want under control?

- As head of this department, have I given all of my key personnel a focus for accomplishing their goals?

- Prior to meeting with the executive director of the hospital and committing my department to a goal-setting procedure, have I clearly examined all of my plans for my key personnel with regard to goals?

- Do I have all of their ideas squared away?

These questions are important to ask because goals should be defined as to the amount and direction of change that is desired in a given period of time. This can begin with an analysis of the current need status of the department and hospital. This type of auditing may be referred to as a needs analysis. The needs analysis examines four issues:

1. What is the basic purpose of the health care institution?
2. What are its strengths?
3. What are its weaknesses?
4. What trends should be envisioned in important key areas?

The examination of weaknesses and strengths that has just been suggested will help the administrator look at objectives that should be immediately established to overcompensate for the weaknesses, whereas an audit of the strengths will give the administrator a standard method of evaluation to deal with the weaknesses.

Goal setting is clearly a component and essential ingredient of the MBO process. Most experts agree that goals and objectives should be specific and that they should be defined in terms of measurable results. Also, individual and organizational goals should be linked in order to ensure congruency and satisfaction. In an Academy of Management survey (McConkie, 1979, p. 32), selected experts in the field of MBO were asked to look at the goal-setting process as a component of MBO and indicate what characteristics they felt were the most essential to it. In order of priority these were:

1. Goals and objectives should be specific.
2. Goals and objectives should be defined in terms of measurable results.
3. Individual goals should be linked to overall organizational goals.
4. Objectives should be reviewed periodically.
5. The time period for goal accomplishment should be specified.
6. Wherever possible, the indicator of the results should be quantifiable; otherwise, it should be at least verifiable.
7. Objectives should be flexible and changed as conditions warrant.
8. Objectives should include a plan of action for accomplishing the results.
9. Objectives should be assigned priorities of weight.

The major authorities whose theories were congruent with this goal-setting process as reviewed in the literature were Peter Drucker, Douglas McGregor, Rensis Likert, George Odiorne, Bert Scanlan, Henry Tosi and Stephen Carroll, Harry Levison, William Reddin, Harold Koontz, John Humble, Tony Raia, and Glenn Varney. The experts also suggested that heavy subordinate involvement in the goal-setting process is essential and they felt subordinates should set goals and present them to top management to review, critique, and approve. They also indicated that superiors and subordinates could jointly set goals, and finally, that there could be some combination of these two processes which would be effective and efficient. These experts also agreed that objective criteria and performance standards must be clearly included in the MBO process or the ensuing appraisal process will be a problem. The consensus of MBO experts seemed to be that where performance is measured, performance improves (McConkie, p. 33).

## CHARACTERISTICS OF HOSPITAL GOALS

Hospital goals should have certain characteristics and requirements to achieve maximum effectiveness and meaningfulness. They should be (Bennett, 1978, pp. 90-91):

- *Balanced and extensive.* Hospital goals should provide a balance in the recognition of a variety of areas where improved performance and results are vital to the future growth and development of the total enterprise. A balanced coverage of multiple goals should be designed and documented to maximize the extent to which managers at all levels and in all areas of hospital operation can identify their relationship and contribution to the hospital goals. Critical areas of coverage requiring consideration include: responsibility to community and patient; human resources, management and nonmanagement employees; financial resources; physical resources; productivity and profitability; and new and innovative developments.

- *Directed toward measurement.* Hospital goals, where possible, should be expressed in such a way as to establish measurable expectations.

- *Present-oriented and future-oriented.* Hospital goals should provide, where appropriate, long-range goals (three to five years) to which the goals for the year ahead can be related. Thus, the goal-setting process requires thinking about the future. However, basic to a consideration of a mission for the organization in the future is a clear recognition of how well the organization is doing right now.

- *Designed for guidance.* The primary role of hospital goals is to provide guidance and direction to all levels of management in the setting of objectives and the planning of action, which contribute to the success of the enterprise. Thus, the collection of hospital goals should possess clarity, be broad in scope, and be based on a careful determination of the real needs of the organization, as well as on an identification of priorities with respect to those needs.

- *In touch with the environment.* Hospitals goals should go beyond a recognition of the need for continuity in the traditional sense and should reflect an awareness and sensitivity to changes (actual and probable) occurring in the external environment of the hospital. Thus, the goals should provide opportunities for innovation and should not be fully introspective in nature. The hospital goals need to answer the question "What are we trying to achieve and become?" and, in so doing, should clearly represent value systems people believe in. Internal considerations, on the other hand, should be based on an analysis of corporate strengths and weaknesses, management capabilities, and resources of the institution.

- *Based on consensus.* Although the authorship of the hospital goals document may rest with the executive director and his planning committee, its content should reflect the consensus expressed by the members of the organizational family, whose commitment to the goals is essential.

- *In keeping with the principle of disclosure.* The question of who or what segments or levels of the organization should be privy to the goals of the organization is an inappropriate one to ask. All personnel need to know and understand the goals. The communication of goals and their importance needs to be achieved in two ways: (1) meaningful participation and involvement on the part of hospital personnel in the goal-setting process and (2) continuing communication of goals after their adoption.

- *Focused on results.* Hospital goals should focus on results. Thus, they need to be couched in language that avoids vague generalizations and platitudes and places attention on real and meaningful expectations of organizational achievement. What must be done is to direct the vision and efforts of all managerial employees toward a set of common goals.

- *Subject to continuous monitoring.* There is a need for (1) reviewing the goals constantly to ensure their appropriateness over time and (2) continually examining and evaluating progress being made toward achieving goals.

## MBO CASE STUDY

One of the most effective methods for managing physical, fiscal, human, and time-oriented resources is by the development of an objective-oriented problem-solving blueprint. Appendix 7-A presents a model for a one-year MBO blueprint, describing the development of routine objectives, problem-solving objectives, innovative objectives, and personal objectives by the Manager of Management Services for the Bennett Hospital. Routine objectives are those which are necessary for ongoing performance, while problem-solving objectives are critical for successful performance. Innovative objectives are desirable for improved performance and a bit futuristic, while personal objectives affect the role and career of the individual within the health care organization. This expanded MBO blueprint focuses upon priorities, desired level of performance, key result areas needed, cost-feasibility projections, and time commitments within which these objectives are to be achieved. If this procedure is performed properly, the organization has an excellent managerial control. If it is not, then efficiency and performance are negatively affected, with loss of time as the result.

## PROBLEMS OF MBO

While management by objectives has multiple assets, no system is foolproof. If the new manager is in the position of managing people he is unfamiliar with, or if the individual must work with objectives for jobs he knows very little about, the potential for problems will be great and the total project will be somewhat conflict laden. Many of the problems associated with MBO are often overlooked, as are the limitations of this procedure. MBO is not a panacea, even when it is utilized with maximum effectiveness. Managers waste resources, manpower, and time by not dealing with the bugs in the system.

Levinson (1970), in his article "Management by Whose Objectives?" comments (pp. 125-134):

> Because it is based on a reward/punishment psychology, the process of management by objective in combination with performance appraisal is self-defeating. Moreover, this technique is one of the greatest management illusions, and serves simply to increase pressure on the individual. I do not reject the MBO process itself, but the technique can be improved by examining the underlying assumptions about the motivation, by taking group action, and by considering the individual's personal goals first.

While MBO has a great many assets, it often does create hostility, resentment, and distrust between management and subordinates. It was actually designed to be a fair, impartial, and reasonable process to determine job performance and appraisal. At the same time it was also designed to allow the individual the opportunity to be self-motivated by setting his own objectives. Yet, MBO often begins to do the opposite of what it sets out to do, and that is to take the individual into consideration.

Some organizations may have been initially attracted to the technique by the claimed advantages of MBO and may even have begun establishing such a system without being cognizant of the complex organizational and individual problems that can arise. If some of these problems can be recognized and corrected, the system will be more effective, with a resultant time and effort saving on the part of the health care manager. Some of the problems are:

- A lack of top management support and involvement in the MBO process. This is one of the most frequently mentioned problem areas in management literature. The active involvement and participation of top levels of the health care organization is vital to the perpetuation of the entire MBO process. Therefore, individual objectives must be set in conjunction with the next higher level in the organizational hierarchy as described by Drucker. It is crucial that a top-level commitment to MBO be given since this is a necessary ingredient for protection against failure.

- If the MBO program operating within the organization is characterized by being highly centralized with regard to decision making and an authoritarian operation, then the program will probably fail. The individuals within the organization, both managers and subordinates alike, must be permitted to fully participate in the program to the extent that their contributions are being used. With preestablished goals, little weight can be given to areas of creativity for the individual, which often becomes demotivating and inhibiting. In too many cases, top management establishes the goals for the organization and then leaves it to run itself. At a later date, these managers cannot understand why the program has failed. The fact that MBO brings along with it organizational change is probably one of the most important reasons why top-management commitment and control are needed.

- Managers must develop skills in identifying and establishing key performance objectives and must have the ability to express them in clear and precise terms. Expertise in coaching and counselling and in giving and receiving feedback is also essential. These managers need a great deal of training to understand the requirements of MBO and their personal involvement in it. Unfortunately, organizations do not believe in development, seeing it as a cost and not an investment. The manpower and time which is lost by this practice creates abundant problems for administrators of MBO.

- Another stumbling block for MBO is the failure to reward performance, since the connection between rewards and performance in MBO is not always made entirely clear. Many managers mistakenly feel that MBO is a process that is isolated from the actual compensation of the employee. A recommendation would be to link performance to rewards. This concern can be explored by looking at issues such as the quality of health care, and the quantity of effort expended in a job, and the available monies for departments who are considered to be effective and efficient and for those managers who successfully fulfill their objectives. This is dependent upon the organization performing an analytical determination of the nature of jobs and their value to the organization. Hopefully, this will replace the all too often competitive systems developed by institutions as solutions to these problems.

- One of the most critical problems of MBO is the conflict between organizational and personal objectives. Most MBO processes concentrate primarily on stated and known organizational objectives and too often ignore individual personal goals. If both objectives are in conflict, then the individual may be forced to compromise his personal values in favor of organizational objectives or leave the organization and pursue his own objectives elsewhere. Therefore, an MBO system must consider personal objectives with the same importance as organizational objectives. The congruence of both results in a symbiotic relationship mutually beneficial to both partners.

- Another problem that occurs frequently in MBO is the manager having to achieve a goal for which he must rely on others within the interdependent system or being staffed with personnel over whom he has no control. To avoid this problem, the MBO program management should encourage team-building processes. This recommendation would take into consideration group goal setting and group evaluations based on group performance. The value of this is to protect the individual against being castigated for making an individual mistake within a group climate. This procedure would permit the manager to control his goals more completely, based upon group value systems.

- One other problem to consider is deciding who should set the objectives. Rather than trust subordinates to develop appropriate and meaningful objectives for themselves, all too often managers dictate the objectives to be set as they want them, with no opportunity for compromise or mutual agreement. This autocratic objective-setting process is programmed for failure since the goal setter must understand the end result for which he is responsible and how this contributes to the total organizational objective.

- Another issue that is equally a problem for the MBO process is the difficulty in measuring and quantifying the goals to be achieved in the process. Certain health care positions and their respective performance criteria are difficult to measure and quantify. This may be due to the nature of the job, lack of data, or lack of experience with goal orientation. If this is the case, management should stress the MBO process and system and not the specific objective itself. As time goes by, individuals involved will become more proficient in developing the MBO components around quantifiable information. It will then actually be their vested system.

- MBO tends to become a one-to-one personal process which often creates a split in the unit's team approach, resulting in other problems. The one-to-one approach does not take into account the interdependent nature of most jobs within a system nor does it ensure the optimal consideration of objectives. One of the advantages of MBO is that there is synchronized integration of the objectives for all managers in the work unit. The responsibility for this type of coordination is left entirely to the manager since he is the only individual in the process who has formal contact with the network of subordinates. One-to-one interaction often becomes a problem when it does not encourage maximum coordination for improvement in superior and subordinate relationships. Research has found that after an intensive and carefully planned MBO program that emphasized subordinate participation, most managers did not feel that the relationship between the two improved. This is a major consideration in looking at MBO and some of its flaws.

- MBO is a solid and lucid indicator of the effectiveness of top- and middle-level management. Without guidelines and guidance from the top, the organizational mission may become suboptimized and diluted. This MBO failure and change in the organization may cause resentment on the part of the managers who were forced into the procedure and who may also feel the process is being forced upon them without a true top-level commitment. Top-level management must also provide support and direction for the program so that all subordinate managers understand what their respective roles are to be in the overall process.

- The overemphasizing of MBO at the expense of other tasks is another problem. There is a danger of being ''MBO obsessive'' to the point where an individual may overlook other essential aspects of his job or may pursue his own objectives at the expense of the total organization. This then becomes another problem of suboptimization. A manager may make a decision which in the short run appears to be beneficial, but in the long run may become a problem. It is important in this case for the manager to always discuss the subordinate's goals and the organization's goals to determine if there is some degree of congruence. The important point to consider is that although needs should be compatible between both parties, personal goals should never be met at the expense of the organization. In the final analysis, management must lead.

- An example of overemphasizing the MBO commitment is a health care manager stating within his own MBO charter that he expects to cut costs within his department by 20 percent at the end of the year. To accomplish this he may decide not to hire additional personnel in his department, which would decrease his costs but also reduce the quality of health care. This short-range judgment often defeats the best-intentioned MBO effort and leads to failure and wasted time.

- If objectives are set too quickly while the program is perceived as new and faddish, there may not be enough interaction between the different levels of the organization to actualize the elements of the program. When this occurs, the objectives appear to have been thrown together superficially and too quickly. This demonstrates a lack of teamwork and control and the program now becomes another headache in need of a solution. This situation will become time-consuming and resource draining.

- There are other objectives that tend to present difficulties in implementation and measurement—those that attempt to cover more than one function. For example, the financial and the human resource departments in the hospital could very well develop a joint MBO to develop a compensation and wage and salary program. It must be clearly defined which departments will perform what tasks and by what date. The problem that may occur is that if one department (financial) does perform as initially committed, the total objective cannot be fully achieved if the other department (human resources) fails to perform its component within the MBO process. The manager who reviews this situation must analyze and evaluate the performance of each individual within the MBO process in this example since it is not equitable to hold the second department (human resources) responsible for the primary department's (financial) failure, even though the total MBO procedure was not accomplished. It is crucial for management to diagnose and dissect those functions in a multidisciplinary approach in which team objectives are perceived by management as being significant. Currently, more and more objectives are being formulated as interfunctional objectives because organizations are beginning to utilize a total systems approach to management which encompasses multifunction planning.

- Another problem in the MBO process is that of poorly conducted performance appraisal reviews, which can undermine the total MBO program. Most appraisal and review systems are based upon a simple checklist of redundant criteria that requires little real effort on the part of the reviewer. If the evaluation system is nebulous and performance standards are vague, the procedure will suffer from either the "halo" effect or the "horns." In the "halo effect," preconceived notions lead to rating an employee in a most favorable manner, either because of the manager's rigid perceptions of past performance, compatibility with others, or a "no complaint" bias. In the "horns effect," individuals are rated extremely low, perhaps because the supervisor is a perfectionist, or because the personality patterns of both are in conflict. Needless to say, evaluations based on criteria that are not so subjective are recommended.

- The misuse of MBO as a punitive device is a problem. MBO has been misused by managers in attempting to control their subordinates and by not getting commitment from subordinates on goals that the subordinate alone must achieve. Without consultation with his subordinate, the manager is in total control and therefore abuses the MBO system. The purpose of MBO is to have both parties contribute to the process. There is always the danger that goals will become obsolete through change or unforeseen events, and the MBO system must be flexible enough (contingency approach) to allow the individual to adjust his MBO program to these events by working with his manager. When the manager resists making changes to the MBO and informs his subordinate that the agreement has already been established and "written in concrete," it generates resistance to MBO and becomes an extremely negative control device. Subordinates usually try to sabotage the efforts of their managers when they are backed into a corner in this manner.

- Managerial obsolescence is an important problem to consider in the MBO process. Managers who are in midcareer may not have been exposed to MBO and its ramifications as junior executives or college students. By not being aware of the latest trends and systems of management science, these managers often find MBO or any innovative system to be extremely difficult to accept and comprehend. They find the system threatening and only view this process as an imposed fad and not as an integrative element to be incorporated within their system.

- There is also the obsession with time and "deadlineitis!" For some reason, MBO seems to be absurdly tied by management directly to a calendar or fiscal year. This connotes that once a year an organization will enumerate what its objectives will be for the forthcoming year. This is even done when organizations are cognizant of the contingencies and opportunities that can happen at any time. Therefore, the MBO system should be performance and results oriented and not related to a time element. It appears to be natural to set goals for short periods of time of less than a year, or even quarterly. Based on this rationale and the dynamic changes within organizations, there is no reason for goals to be set for the long run when short-run results are less difficult to establish and evaluate. One of the problems, however, is that organizations seem to need time periods for evaluation and appraisal which directly affect their computer, compensation systems, fiscal periods and top management's personal idiosyncrasies.

- Managers create paperwork dilemmas by becoming overly involved with the unnecessary and often abundant paperwork generated by MBO. This paperwork actually becomes the end result and the MBO system only serves as the means. A successful system should be simple and as relatively free of redundant paperwork as possible. The only area where paperwork should be involved is where it is essential.

- Managers often confuse total results with quantifiable results of MBO. This overemphasis on numbers is one of the major problems of the program. Such thinking forces individuals to avoid the objectives that cannot be quantified in the short run. A different type of verification is required so that qualitative aspects of the process are considered as well. It is essential to have a system in which complex objectives tend to be produced as hedges against unsatisfactory performance. It is the manager's responsibility to develop and support a realistic approach to the objective setting of his subordinates.

These problems with MBO do have a number of solutions which can be considered in the quest to make this system as viable and effective as it can optimally be. The MBO process as presented throughout this chapter and in the Chapter Appendix case study is a most realistic technique and theory to employ as a resource for actualizing organizational goals and saving that valuable resource—time.

## REFERENCES

Appelbaum, S.H. An experiential case study of organizational suboptimization and problem solving. *Akron Business and Economic Review,* Fall 1975, *6*(3), 13.

Bennett, A.C. Effective managers must have both vision and purpose. *Hospitals–JAHA,* April 1976, *50,* 67.

Bennett, A.C. *Improving management performance in health care institutions: A total systems approach.* Chicago: American Hospital Association, 1978.

Carroll, S.J., & Tosi, H.L., Jr. *Management by objectives: Applications and research.* New York: Macmillan Co., 1973.

Conley, W.D., & Miller, F.W. MBO, pay and productivity. *Personnel,* January/February 1973, *50,* 21-25.

Cyert, R.M., & March, J.G. Organizational goals. In *A behavioral theory of the firm.* Englewood Cliffs, N.J.: Prentice Hall, 1963, Ch. III.

Deegan, A.X., II. *Management by objectives for hospitals.* Germantown, Md.: Aspen Systems Corp. 1977.

Deniston, O.L., Rosenstock, I.M., & Getting, V.A. Evaluation of program effectiveness. *Public Health Reports,* April 1968, *83,* 323-335.

Donabedian, A. *Aspects of medical care administration: Specifying requirements for health care.* Cambridge, Mass.: Harvard University Press, 1973.

Drucker, P.F. *The practice of management.* New York: Harper and Row, 1954.

Drucker, P.F. *People and performance: The best of Peter Drucker on management.* New York: Harper Press, 1977.

Du Bois, D.M. Organizational viability of group practice. *Group Practice,* April 1967, *16,* 8-9.

Ford, R.C., & Bell, R.R. MBO: Seven strategies for success. *S.A.M. Advanced Management Journal,* Winter 1977, 14-24.

Gordon, G.C., & Goldberg, B.E. Is there a climate for success? *Management Review,* May 1977, *66* (5), 41.

Hand, H., & Hollingsworth, A.T. Tailoring MBO to hospitals. In A.M. Glassman (Ed.), *The challenge of management.* New York: John Wiley and Sons, 1978.

Herzlinger, R. Can we control health care costs? *Harvard Business Review,* March-April 1978, *56*(2), 102-110.

Hollingsworth, A.T., & Mobley, W.H. Relationships among individual variables, organizational variables, performance and attrition in hospitals. *Proceedings of the 38th Annual Meeting of the Academy of Management,* August 1978, 348-350.

Kelly, J. *How managers manage.* Englewood Cliffs, N.J.: Prentice Hall, 1980.

Kiev, A. *A strategy for handling executive stress.* Chicago: Nelson Hall, 1974.

Latham, G.P., & Yukl, G.A. A review of research on the application of goal setting in organizations. *Academy of Management Journal,* December 1975, *18*(4), 824-845.

Levinson, H. Management by whose objectives? *Harvard Business Review,* July-August 1970, *48*(4), 125-134.

Likert, R. *The human organization.* New York: McGraw-Hill Book Co., 1967.

Locke, E.A. Personnel attitudes and motivation. *Annual Review of Psychology,* 1975, *26,* 457-480.

Locke, E.A., & Bryan, J.F. Performance goals as determinants of level of performance and boredom. *Journal of Applied Psychology,* April 1967, *51,* 120-130.

McConkey, D. *How to manage by results*. New York: American Management Association, 1965.

McConkie, M.L. A clarification of the goal setting and appraisal process in MBO. *Academy of Management Review,* April 1979, *4*(1), 29-40.

Meglino, B.M. Stress and performance: Implications for organizational policies. *Supervisory Management,* April 1977, *22,* 22-28.

Mitchell, T.R. *People in organizations: Understanding their behavior*. New York: McGraw-Hill Book Co., 1978, 318.

Raia, A.P. *Managing by objectives*. Glenview, Ill.: Scott, Foresman and Co., 1974, 29.

Scheff, T.J. Differential displacement of treatment goals in a mental hospital. *Administrative Science Quarterly,* September 1962, *7,* 208-217.

Simon, H.A. *Administrative behavior*. New York: Macmillan & Co., 1961, 62-66.

Appendix 7-A

# Objectives for the Management Systems Engineering Department, Bennett Hospital for Fiscal Year 1981*

## INTRODUCTION

This is the first report presenting objectives for the Management Systems Engineering Department (MSED). These objectives will be initiated or attained during fiscal year 1981. Status reports on the attainment of these objectives will be developed on a quarterly basis commencing in October, 1980.

These objectives support the objectives of the Materials and Management Services Division, dated April 26, 1980, as prepared by Derek R. Ford, Director of Materials and Management Services.

The following two factors were considered during the development of the objectives presented in this report:

1. The decision to add the Management Systems Engineering (MSE) Department to the Hospital's Table of Organization was made in the Fall of 1979. The Department became operational in January, 1978. Thus, the MSED is a "new" organizational function.
2. Although the Hospital had previously used MSE services on a consulting basis, the services were not organized to provide continuous support.

In view of the above factors, the types of services provided by the MSED will not be constrained by any objectives which may have been established prior to the inception of the current Department.

---

*Presented by Ralph B. Turner, Manager of Management Services to Derek R. Ford, Director of Materials and Management Services, September, 1980.

While reviewing these objectives, note that the MSED is a staff function and, as such, can only recommend changes which serve to achieve the objectives of the Hospital. The various functions within the Hospital have the primary responsibility for implementing approved recommendations. This discussion does not apply to those objectives which are solely within the control of the MSED.

## SUMMARY OF ROUTINE OBJECTIVES

The following Key Result Areas (KRA) were identified for the MSED:

KRA No. 1:   Project Services
KRA No. 2:   Project Management
KRA No. 3:   MSE Program Management

For each of these KRAs, several methods of measurement were identified and are detailed on the following pages. The identification of priorities is not required for Routine Objectives.

**Routine Objectives**

| Key Result Area | As Measured by | Present Level | Desired Level |
|---|---|---|---|
| 1. Project Services | (a) Number of new project requests | | (a) 1-2 per month (3-month average) |
| | (b) Number of completed projects | | (b) 1 every 2 months (6-month average) |
| | (c) Savings in dollars | | (c) 1.5 to 1.0 return on the MSED resource (cumulative total for year) |
| | (d) Level of service/quality | | (d) 10-25% improvement over existing level (6-month average) |
| | (e) Percent billable services | | (e) For Senior MSE: Monthly Average of 82% For MSE: Monthly Average of 84% |
| 2. Project Management | (a) Percent variance in resource budget | | (a) 0 - 20% greater than budget per project |
| | (b) Percent variance in completion schedules | | (b) 0 - 40% behind schedule per project |
| | (c) Project status reports | | (c) As required by the project work plan |
| | (d) Project team meeting | | (d) Evidence of compatible working relationship and 0 -1 complaints per month total for all active projects |

| 3. MSE Program | (a) | MSE program status reports | (a) | As required by MSE Table 1C, current revision, and evidence of satisfactory feedback from Director of Materials and Management Services |
| | (b) | Status meetings with the director of Materials and Management Services | (b) 1 per week | (b) 1 per week |

### SUMMARY OF PROBLEM-SOLVING OBJECTIVES

The following listing corresponds to the problem-solving objectives (PSO) detailed on the following pages. Once these PSOs are approved, and the solution options selected, work plans will be developed and submitted to the Director of Materials and Management Services Department for approval.

- Key result area: *Program Management*                                     *Priority*

    PSO No. 1:  Communications between the                      A
    MSED and the top management staff are
    not as effective as they could be.

    PSO No. 2:  A mechanism for requesting                      C
    the services of the MSED does not cur-
    rently exist. Supports Objective #30 of the
    M&MSD.

- Key result area: *Project Management*

    PSO No. 3:  There are too many projects                     B
    incurring negative variances in completion
    schedules.

    PSO No. 4:  Projects being performed by                     A
    internal and external consultants are not
    being managed in a ''consistent'' manner
    and status reporting on same is not done on
    a formal basis. Supports Objective #30 of
    the M&MSD.

## Problem-Solving Objective No. 1

*Statement of Problem*

Communications between the MSED and the top management staff are not as effective as they could be.

*Present Status*

Bi-monthly MSE Program Status Reports are distributed to the top management staff. Three (3) status reports have been distributed during the period from January through May, 1980. Individual or group review meetings have not been held to review these reports. There has been no feedback received on these reports.

*Desired Status*

Direct face-to-face communications between the MSED and the top management staff should support the material presented in these reports.

*Basis for Desired Status*

Face-to-face communications are necessary for the achievement of complete communication.

*Examination of Causes*

1. Management style of CEO—apparently the CEO prefers "on demand" face-to-face meetings with his subordinates rather than scheduled meetings attended by all of his subordinates.
2. Hospital Management Environment—apparently management planning, control, and reporting are handled on an informal basis, i.e., management reports are not prepared and formal evaluation meetings to review progress on current assignments are not held.
3. MSE Program Status Reports do not address the informational requirements of the top management staff.

| | Criteria | | |
|---|---|---|---|
| *Options* | *Contribution to Objective* | *Cost* | *Feasibility* |
| 1. Meet face-to-face with each top manager on an individual basis. | Medium | Medium | High |
| 2. Meet face-to-face with all of the top managers on a group basis. | Medium | Medium | Medium |
| 3. Perform a survey to assess the information requirements of the top management staff. | High | Medium | High |
| 4. Design and coordinate the implementation of an MSE Steering Committee (would impact PSO No. 2 also). | High | High | Low |
| Ideal | High | Low | High |

## Problem-Solving Objective No. 2

*Statement of Problem*

A mechanism for requesting the services of the MSED does not currently exist.

*Present Status*

The director of Materials and Management Services refers, approves, and schedules new projects. A procedure for requesting a project study does not exist nor has the responsibility for approving and scheduling new projects been assigned under the current system.

*Desired Status*

A procedure should exist detailing how a project request is submitted, how it is processed and by whom and at what step decisions are made.

*Basis for Desired Status*

In order to fully evaluate the demand for the services of the MSED, a mechanism should exist to facilitate access to these services.

In addition, for the complete acceptance of the services of the MSED, cost center managers should be able to access these services via a standard operating procedure. Without an access mechanism, the MSED could be viewed as an "espionage" function working for the top management staff.

*Examination of Causes*

1. Hospital organization climate—management priorities change rapidly; a procedural mechanism would tend to inhibit the processing rate of these changes.
2. Cost Center managers are not knowledgeable of the services provided by the MSED.
3. Resistance of the director of Materials and Management Services—implementation of a mechanism would erode some of his control over the allocation of the services of the MSED.

| | Criteria | | |
| --- | --- | --- | --- |
| *Options* | *Contribution to Objective* | *Cost* | *Feasibility* |
| 1. Reassess the rate of change in priorities. | Medium | Low | Low |

| | | | |
|---|---|---|---|
| 2. Implement an MSE marketing program for cost center managers. | High | Medium | Medium |
| 3. Develop and implement a project request and approval procedure (would also support PSO No. 1). | High | Medium | Medium |
| Ideal | High | Low | High |

## Problem-Solving Objective No. 3

*Statement of Problem*

There are too many projects incurring a negative variance in completion schedules.

*Present Status*

Several projects exceeding the planned completion date by more than 50 percent (subjective estimate).

*Desired Status*

Maximum of 40 percent variance in completion schedules (assuming no change in project scope).

*Basis for Desired Status*

Experience has indicated that this is an achievable and desirable standard of performance for an internal consulting service. Achievement of this standard will normally be acceptable to the project clients.

*Examination of Causes*

1. Estimating ability of MSE staff.

2. Change in project priorities.

3. Individual staff members assigned too many active projects.

**Criteria**

| Options | Contribution to Objective | Cost | Feasibility |
|---------|---------------------------|------|-------------|
| 1. Project management education for MSE. staff. | Low | High | High |
| 2. Develop a six-month project plan. | High | High | Medium |
| 3. Determine a standard for the number of active projects per staff member. | Medium | Low | Medium |
| Ideal | High | Low | High |

## Problem-Solving Objective No. 4

*Statement of Problem*

Projects being performed by internal and external consultants are not being managed in a "consistent" manner and status reporting on same is not done on a formal basis.

*Present Status*

The director of Materials and Management Services is responsible for the management of both internal and external consultants. The MSED is the only function which develops a written report concerning the status of active projects as measured against the "plan" for each project. A single report indicating the status of all the currently assigned projects is not developed.

*Desired Status*

One report should be developed reporting on the status of all active projects.

*Basis for Desired Status*

Written status reports support the management of the achievement of project objectives.

*Examination of Causes*

1. Lack of a formal mechanism for the management of services provided by consulting resources.
2. Management style of the director of Materials and Management Services.
3. Numerous reporting relationships for the various consulting resources.

**Criteria**

| Options | Contribution to Objective | Cost | Feasibility |
|---|---|---|---|
| 1. Develop a formal mechanism for the management of the services provided by consulting resources (relates to PSO No. 1 and No. 2). | Medium | Medium | Medium |
| 2. Restructure the job of the Director of Materials and Management Services. | Medium | Low | Medium |
| 3. Have all consulting resources managed by the MSED. | High | High | Medium |
| Ideal | High | Low | High |

## SUMMARY OF PROBLEM-SOLVING OBJECTIVES

The following listing corresponds to the Innovative Objectives (IO) detailed on the following pages. Once these IOs are approved, detailed proposals will be developed and submitted to the director of Materials and Management Services for approval.

*Priority*

IO No. 1: Develop and implement a Forms Management     C
Program. Supports Objective No. 27 of the
M&MSD.

IO No. 2: Develop and implement a Materials Control     B
Program. Supports Objective No. 28 of the
M&MSD.

IO No. 3: Determine the feasibility of implementing a          B
           Production Planning Control System. Supports
           Objective No. 19 and No. 26 of the M&MSD.

IO No. 4: Determine the feasibility of centralizing the         A
           Quality Assurance Program. Supports Objective
           No. 7 of the M&MSD.

## Innovative Objective No. 1

*Description*

Develop and implement a Forms Management Program.

*Desired Results*

1. Reduction of total forms material costs by 25 percent during the first two years following implementation.
2. Reduction of the total number of forms used by 15 percent during the first two years following implementation.
3. Reduction in forms processing costs of 15 percent during the first two years following implementation.

*Approach*

1. Evaluate the current forms management system and report findings.
   Calendar time requirements: 4-8 weeks
2. Develop recommendations which will support the achievement of the above desired results.
   Calendar time requirements: 4-8 weeks
3. Implement the recommendations.
   Calendar time requirements: 4-12 weeks
4. Evaluate the actual results vs. the desired results and report findings.
   Calendar time requirements: Every 3 months following the completion of the implementation of the recommendations; reference No. 3 above.

## Innovative Objective No. 2

*Description*

Develop and implement a Materials Control Program.

*Desired Results*

1. Reduction of total cost of materials by 10 percent during the first two years following implementation.

2. Existence within 4 months after proposal of a closed loop system for controlling the addition, deletion, or revision of materials.
3. Existence within one year following implementation of design and quality specifications for all materials that are administered to or come in contact with patients.

*Approach*

1. Evaluate the current materials control system and report findings.
   Calendar time requirements: 4-8 weeks
2. Develop recommendations which will support the achievement of the above desired results.
   Calendar time requirements: 4-8 weeks
3. Implement the recommendations.
   Calendar time requirements: 4-16 weeks
4. Evaluate the actual results vs. the desired results and report findings.
   Calendar time requirements: Every 3 months following the completion of the implementation of the recommendations; reference No. 3 above.

## Innovative Objective No. 3

*Description*

Determine the feasibility of implementing a Production Planning and Control System.

*Desired Results*

1. Reduction in the variability of the average monthly census by 10 percent within one year following implementation.
2. Ability to forecast the workload demand volumes for both direct and indirect patient care functions. Once the workload demand volumes have been forecasted, optimal staff levels can be determined.
3. Existence within two years following implementation of resource requirement specifications for those inpatient services which represent 80 percent of the total service demand.

*Approach*

1. Evaluate the current inpatient admissions scheduling system and report findings.
   Calendar time requirements: 4-8 weeks

2. Evaluate the current ancillary services scheduling systems and report findings.
   Calendar time requirements: 6-12 weeks
3. Develop a system for forecasting workload demand.
   Calendar time requirements: 4-8 weeks
4. Develop new scheduling systems which will support the achievement of the above desired results.
   Calendar time requirements: 8-12 weeks
5. Implement the system for forecasting workload demand.
   Calendar time requirements: 4-6 weeks
6. Implement the new scheduling systems.
   Calendar time requirements: 8-16 weeks
7. Evaluate the actual results vs. the desired results and report findings.
   Calendar time requirements: Every 3 months following the completion of the above two implementation phases; reference No. 5 and No. 6 above.

## Innovative Objective No. 4

*Description*

Determine the feasibility of centralizing the hospital's Quality Assurance Program (QAP). This study would include a review of the following existing functions:

| | |
|---|---|
| Utilization review | Patient advocate |
| Infection control | Medical records |
| Tissue pathology | Bio-medical engineering (contracted) |

This objective will support the maintenance of the Quality-Productivity Management System scheduled for implementation during the Winter of 1980-81.

*Desired Results*

1. Centralization of the QAP within the hospital's table of organization.
2. Measurement of the return on investment on the hospital's current (QAP) within 6 months following the implementation of the recommendations developed during this study.
3. Evidence of improved management of the hospital's QAP within one year following the implementation of the recommendations developed during this study.

4. Implementation of an integrated hospital-wide quality assurance system which would quantitatively measure the performance of the various hospital systems vs. quality engineered standards.
5. A return on investment of 15 percent within two years following the implementation of a centralized, integrated, and engineered QAP.

*Approach*

1. Evaluate the current organization of the QAP and report findings.
   Calendar time requirements: 4-8 weeks
2. Estimate the effectiveness of the current QAP.
   Calendar time requirements: 4-8 weeks
3. Develop recommendations for the centralization of the QAP.
   Calendar time requirements: 4-6 weeks
4. Implement these recommendations.
   Calendar time requirements: 4-6 weeks
5. Design a new quality assurance system.
   Calendar time requirements: 6-12 weeks
6. Develop quality engineered standards for this system.
   Calendar time requirements: 1-3 years
7. Implement the new quality assurance system.
   Calendar time requirements: 1-3 years
8. Evaluate the actual results vs. the desired results and report findings.
   Calendar time requirements: Every 3 months following the completion of the implementation of the recommendations; reference No. 4 above.

## SUMMARY OF PERSONAL DEVELOPMENT OBJECTIVES

The following listing corresponds to the Personal Development Objectives (PDO) detailed on the following pages. These objectives are to be achieved by the author of this report.

|  |  | *Priority* |
|---|---|---|
| PDO No. 1: | Participate in an MBA or MS program majoring in business and finance. | A |
| PDO No. 2: | Participate in the management of the Delaware Shore Hospital Management Engineering Society. | A |
| PDO No. 3: | Publish one professional article or paper in a trade journal or magazine. Supports Objective No 40 of the M&MSD. | B |

PDO No. 4:    Participate as a provider member in Health        C
              Systems Agency representing Burlington
              County, New Mexico.

## Personal Development Objective No. 1

*Description*

Participate in an MBA or MS Program majoring in business and finance.

*Reason for This Objective*

To increase my management knowledge and skills, thereby enhancing my ability to achieve the following career goal within two years: To create the position of Director of Management Services and to be promoted to same.

- Management systems engineering
- Quality assurance, including engineering and inspection, reference Innovative Objective No. 4.
- Forms management program, reference Innovative Objective No. 1.
- Systems management program.

*Time and Action Plan*

1. Select course of study and college or university to attend.
   Schedule: By the end of September, 1980.
2. Begin first semester.
   Schedule: January, 1981.
3. Complete program.
   Schedule: By the end of May, 1985.

## Personal Development Objective No. 2

*Description*

Participate in the management of the Delaware Shore Hospital Management Engineering Society.

*Reason for This Objective*

To gain personal recognition from my peers and to keep abreast of the market for the services of hospital management systems engineers.

*Time and Action Plan*

1. Obtain appointment as a member of the board of directors and as the chairman of the newsletter committee.
Schedule: Completed July, 1980.
2. Publish six issues of the society's newsletter.
Schedule: Bi-monthly, commencing August, 1980.
3. Obtain nomination to the position of president.
Schedule: By February, 1981.

## Personal Development Objective No. 3

*Description*

Publish one professional article or paper in a trade journal or magazine.

*Reason for This Objective*

To gain personal recognition from my peers and from the hospital community which will support the achievement of my current career goal, reference PDO No. 1.

*Time and Action Plan*

1. Identify a topic for publication.
Schedule: By the end of October, 1980.
2. Draft an outline for review.
Schedule: By the end of November, 1980.
3. Select a journal or magazine.
Schedule: By December, 1980.
4. Submit draft for publication.
Schedule: By the end of February, 1981.

## Personal Development Objective No. 4

*Description*

Participate as a provider member in the Health Systems Agency (HSA) representing Burlington County, New Mexico.

*Reason for This Objective*

To gain personal recognition from community leaders and to obtain an understanding of how the HSA accomplishes its mission.

*Time and Action Plan*

1. Register as a member of the HSA.
   Schedule: By the end of September, 1980.
2. Attend three meetings of the HSA Governing Board.
   Schedule: By the end of June, 1981.

# Chapter 8

# The Management of Stress

## TIME MANAGEMENT HIGHLIGHTS

1. Maintenance of an organization is an exercise in existing, while managing is a process characterized as alive and progressing.
2. Psychological-physiological components of stress include coronary disease, occupational stress, coping, stress on the family, stress on the health care manager, and nursing.
3. Managerial-organizational components of stress include health care management, occupational medicine, the troubled employee, managing conflict, managing time, and management by objectives.
4. The scarcity of resources creates anxiety for the health care manager who must decide upon allocations, professional issues, and survival decisions.
5. Wear and tear on the individual under stress and caught in the organizational bind may not only involve progressive damage to the system, but in extreme forms, may result in the actual breakdown and disintegration of the individual and organization.
6. The primary stressor that gives rise to time anxiety is the deadline. This time stress has its own unique problems. Individuals often feel desperate, trapped, and helpless.
7. The patterns of upward mobility at any cost in these organizations lead to neurotic systems often too advanced to manage the unresolved conflicts. This activity needs to be controlled in order to reduce the stressors.
8. Many health care managers create their own stress by assuming extra responsibilities, failing to assign minor tasks to subordinates, or neglecting to insist on realistic deadlines. Appropriate delegation of authority to competent subordinates can ease the burden of overwork and yield some time off.

9. One of the most common situations producing fear, stress, and anxiety for the health care manager is change, which is often a disruption of the status quo and ongoing relationships. Even changes for the better are perceived as losses in which things are given up for new replacements or systems.

10. The manager who is the Type A personality is intense, demanding of self and others, ambitious, competitive, aggressive, aware of time urgency, restless, and impatient. He is content when battling deadlines and obstacles. There are never enough hours in the day for him to achieve tasks. He has a higher probability of developing coronary heart disease or suffering a fatal coronary during the 35 to 40-year-old age period.

11. When managers work under stress, the quality of their work and efficiency is often affected. They compensate for quality by increasing their energy, tension, and time investment. When they face emotional stress the critical psychological cognitive balance is lost and their normal insightful judgments become fragmented, affecting their performance and wasting valuable time through unreliable decision-making processes.

12. Stress management can be achieved by reversing dysfunctional processes that prove to be on a collision course and also by eliminating identified stressors.

Managers have been conditioned to believe that they can manage just about any operation that is seemingly rational and measurable. The challenge of a complex, dynamic organizational problem is enticing to a professional manager. Risks and uncertainty seem to command great interest on the part of administrators who perceive a commensurate reward. Achievement, beating deadlines, and juggling time appear to be part of their orientation. This drive connotes the building of stress—which is more difficult to control and manage than many of their activities.

Managing stress, like managing work, is an illusion. Contemporary elixirs often suggested include relaxation, meditation, nutritional changes, vigorous exercise, finishing unfinished business, assertiveness, time management, and total self-management. Yet these solutions have limited usefulness since stress is an integral part of organizational components such as motivation, planning, decision making, and communications. To manage stress is not to eliminate it, but to identify those dynamics creating unresolved conflicts within the organization (Appelbaum, 1980, p. 7). The management of time is one of these sources of stress.

Psychoanalytic thought seems to suggest that all human beings need to have an appropriate degree of time structuring in order to overcome existential anxiety and to gain feelings of assurance and adequacy. Without some sense of the predictability of events in one's surroundings, individuals often become anxious and disoriented. The relative thoroughness with which various people structure their time depends on their early life experiences and "programs," and on the culture in which they operate.

More than any other people on the face of the earth, Americans seem obsessed with time. There is a very old business adage, "Time is money." We say, "Time and tide wait for no man." We speak of "taking time," "saving time," "killing time," "making up for lost time," "having time," "losing time," and "gaining time." The fact that virtually every American home has a clock, that there are clocks in just about every business office, schoolroom, movie theater, shop, restaurant, and church, and even in automobiles and on highway billboards, makes it very difficult for us to visualize a culture that has no clocks and that does not conceive of time as a commodity—a substance that is to be bought, sold, measured, manipulated, and structured (Albrecht, 1979, p. 88).

In the business world, the principal stressor that gives rise to time anxiety is the deadline. This is our traditional way of getting things done effectively. The combination of a person's total workload, the relative severity of the deadlines involved, and his own personal level of reactivity will determine the level of anxiety.

Each employee has a fairly well-defined comfort zone or sense of urgency and time pressure within which he works effectively and gains a sense of accomplishment. Beyond this zone of reasonable time pressure, deadlines threaten, time seems to run out, there is not enough slack time for pressure relief or change of pace, and the individual begins to feel overstressed. Time stress, although physically the same as all other forms of stress, has its own special mental aspects. One feels desperate, trapped, miserable, and often rather helpless. In cases of very high time stress, one can even begin to feel depressed and hopeless. If one cannot step back and look at the situation and narrow down the required accomplishments to something reasonable, then one is caught like a rat in a trap of his own making (Albrecht, 1979, p. 89).

Health care environments are most complex, yet fascinating organizations in which to study the attempt to achieve goals and beat deadlines. Experience shows that most problems are not technical ones but behavioral ones. Administrators who have been professionally trained possess the tools needed to maintain their organizations, but that is not what managing is all about. *Maintenance is existence, while managing is living and progressing.* The functions of a health care manager, namely, planning, organizing, staffing, directing, coordinating, reporting, and budgeting (Wren, 1972, p. 235), cannot be attempted until other factors are anticipated and managed. These contingencies serve to block the valves of the managerial systems of health care organizations because they directly impact upon those administrators responsible for achieving the critical objectives of these institutions while attempting to fulfill the psychological and physiological needs of employees.

## THE MANAGEMENT ENIGMA

The management of organizational stress within the health care organization is an overwhelming challenge to undertake, but one which is essential and achievable. The creation of stress is unfortunately stimulated by encouraging the utilization and adaptation of managerial systems that have limited credibility and unproven track records. Unfortunately, managers of health care systems perpetuate managerial theories and techniques that they were exposed to earlier in their own career orientation and socialization. Since these methods and philosophies were considered to be popular and acceptable to the mentors and professors of these managers, they continue to be emphasized even when it appears the product is unfeasible, counterproductive, and stress producing. A tentative solution in dealing with the management systems employed by the administration of the health care system is to determine effectiveness and impact. The reversal of dysfunctional management-organizational systems is the starting point in developing these institutions to the point where they become more organic in adapting to change and in resolving conflict. If a management technique is creating a stressful situation for individuals, then it must either be stopped or reversed in order to actualize the mission of achieving objectives and fulfilling needs. The key to managing stress in a health care system is to identify the stressor and eliminate it or completely reverse the process until the stress is reduced to a level considered manageable within the organization.

One of the essential problems in need of solution within health care systems is rarely dealt with or confronted—the question of how much change human beings can accept, absorb, and assimilate, and the rate at which they can take it. Can they keep up with the ever-increasing rate of technological change, or is there some point at which the human organism goes to pieces? Can they leave the static ways and static guidelines which have dominated all of their history and adopt the process ways, the continual changingness which must be theirs if they are to survive? (Rogers, 1973, p. 122).

Change and disruption are equally traumatic for managers of health care systems. They have a difficult time juggling the fiscal-physical-human resources of the system since a major fear is to remain static in a turbulent environment. It is equally disastrous to infuse turbulence and change processes into the system based upon the fallacious premise that dynamic organisms are the survivors while mechanistic systems are doomed to fail. Most industrial managers are not entirely comfortable with the dynamic nature of their operation. This approach also forces the health care manager to attempt to emulate the complex industrial system in his operation. The complexities of this interactive connection between the environment and organization should be described as a system, and a system may be defined as a "purposive collection of interacting entities." It consists of a set of elements that are related to each other in such a way that the actions of one element affect the states of and initiate or modify activity in the others. The first step in describing a system is to establish its boundaries—setting out principles by which it can be decided whether some particular entity is an element of the system or not. A system is said to be bounded by the relationship of its entities to a purpose, function, or sphere of activity: If the element is relevant to the attainment of the system's objectives, it is an element of the system (LaPatra, 1975, p. 9).

The health care manager is faced with many uncertainties within these systems which are conflict laden. Activities necessitate action within boundaries that are unrelated to the organization. Many political, economic, social, legal, and cultural constraints may impede operations and frustrate the best managed and planned efforts. For example, the strong economic pressure to control rising health care costs influences the roles of many health care professionals as well as the boundaries between groups. In the future, more problems may arise when traditional lines of authority and task assignments become obscured as perceived supply deficiencies in human resources are met. The relationship between managing health care and occupational-organizational stress is becoming more pronounced, since delivering the service and organizational survival are complex tasks that often are on a collision course under the stimulus of time.

## THE TARGET: HEALTH CARE

Health care managers are often caught in the middle of crosscurrents since they must promote the concept of health as their service and manage the professionals and organizational resources needed to deliver this service. Health is a state of complete physical, mental, and social well-being and is not merely the absence of disease or infirmity. This definition was adopted in 1946 in the original constitution of the World Health Organization (WHO), and draws heavily on the conception given voice a few years earlier by the great historian of medicine, Henry Sigerist (1941, p. 100): "Health is . . . not simply the absence of disease: It is something positive, a joyful attitude toward life, and a cheerful acceptance of the responsibilities that life puts upon the individual." The WHO definition represents, without doubt, the most concerted effort to develop an explicit consensus regarding the meaning of the word health, and yet, as we shall see, it has by no means been universally accepted as a proper definition. It does serve as a foundation for understanding the technical, human, and managerial missions of health care systems. The fact that modern societies, however organized, devote such great resources to health attests to its social importance. . . . Since resources are limited, we must make choices. Health care at some point must be weighed against other social preferences and commitments (Mechanic, 1972, pp. 3-4). In other words, in the real world we must inevitably stop short of attaining the ideal of health for all people, however it may be defined. We can devote our attention to considering the ways in which humans go about the business of protecting and improving their health without concluding what such efforts might entail. The scarcity of health care resources creates further anxieties and stress for the managers of these systems who must arrive at decisions concerning allocation, management, professionalism, and survival.

A paradox faces those who work to deliver health services: At a time when medical knowledge and clinical capability are at an all-time high, so also is dissatisfaction with health care. The dissatisfaction is not expressed merely by a few malcontents. It is real and widespread, and it comes from all quarters—government, consumers, the providers of care, and those who pay for care as third parties (Longest, 1976, p. 1). The problems which fall within the domain of management can create stress that affects the performance of the institution in delivering its service of health care and organizational survival as well. The demands of time create even greater stress.

Sometimes it takes a catastrophic event or perhaps even a brush with death to give a new and fresh perspective to how one uses time. Recently this happened to a very intense health care manager who rushed about, eagerly accepting extra responsibilities far beyond the call of duty. When not at work he actively participated in a variety of clubs and civic organizations. One day, in his haste to attend a meeting for which he was late, he apparently stumbled and fell down a flight of stairs. The accident necessitated long and complex surgical procedures and, because his overall physical condition was not good, there was some question about his recovery and the imposition of severe limitations once he was allowed to return to work. After a long convalescent period he initially went back to his institution on a part-time basis, gradually increasing the length of his workday. Many former duties, particularly those dealing with detailed matters, had been permanently reassigned to others. His job had been restructured so as to be much less intensive and demanding, and rather more concerned with broader problem-solving aspects of managing the institution. This was indeed fortunate, because his personal physician had warned him of the danger of exposure to stress, and this way the number and frequency of stressful situations which he experienced were sharply reduced. As a result of the accident his entire outlook on the allocation and use of time was completely changed. Today, while he sets goals for himself which some may consider to be quite ambitious, he has learned to live less intensely and not to internalize the problems of the hospital. Each day he sets specified periods of time aside to spend with his family or for personal interests—and the important thing is that he really does it. As a result of the accident and a changed attitude and approach to the use of time, he has successfully removed himself, to a large degree, from stressful situations and seems quite satisfied with his new job responsibilities and life in general.

The following clearly demonstrates the impact of time pressures and deadlines that multiply and ultimately affect the performance of the manager:

Almost by its very nature, your managerial job throws you in the midst of time pressures and deadlines. . . . The urgency of deadlines is real; it is even bound up in the word itself, which evokes an image of a line beyond which lies—death! During periods just before deadlines, the pressure builds up rapidly. But once the deadline is met, everyone feels greatly relieved.

It is not uncommon for a manager to experience the pressure of deadlines in such a way as to question whether he is in control of his life or whether his watch and calendar are controlling him. I once heard a chief executive say that the one piece of equipment he owned that he couldn't do without was his watch. If you have ever had to do without your watch for several days or have lost your calendar indicating all of your appointments for the next week, you know just how stress-provoking this can be.. Whenever I ask managers to identify key stressors in their organizational life, time pressures and deadlines are always at the top of the list. So it is evident that time pressures constitute one of the key stressors intrinsic to a job (Yates, 1979, pp. 41-42).

The American Management Association (AMA) also dealt with this problem in the text *Executive Stress,* a survey report which contained the findings of an investigation of how 2,659 AMA members perceived, experienced, and coped with stress. Some of their conclusions concerning stress are particularly relevant to the management of time (Kiev & Kohn, 1979, pp. 2-3):

1. A large majority of respondents reported stressful job conditions at times, but not with any great frequency. The findings indicate that executives who face daily crises, pressures and frustrations are in a minority.
2. Among the factors cited as most stress-producing are work and time pressures, with 73 percent of top level and 71 percent of middle management ranking the two highest.
3. The respondents suggested analyzing the stressful situation and then deciding what is worth worrying about and what should be dismissed as the most effective means of coping with stress.

They also stated (p. 56):

It is important to note that although many managers work for organizations in which high value is placed on productivity and time schedules are tight, it is also true that many managers create their own stress by taking on extra responsibilities, failing to assign ancillary tasks to subordinates, or neglecting to insist on realistic deadlines.

It was suggested that managers must set a pace that will avoid physical and mental fatigue and concomitant stress disorders. With appropriate delegation of authority to competent subordinates, a manager can lighten the burden of overwork and get a little time off to maintain or regain equanimity. Pressures vary with the exigencies of the business, but a manager can set priorities so that the most important goals are reached.

## A PROBLEM OF AND FOR SOCIETY

Stress is considered one of society's most urgent problems. Stress arises when there is a deviation from optimum conditions that the individual cannot easily correct, resulting in an imbalance between demand and capacity. For serious stress to occur, the individual must view as serious the consequences of failure to have demands met. Such a formulation of stress demands that social and environmental conditions, as well as native endowment, training, and bodily conditions, be examined. In short, anything that affects demand or capacity has the potential to produce (or to alleviate) stress.

The "inverted-U" hypothesis informs us that performance improves with increasing arousal, up to a point, when it declines as arousal becomes more than optimal. The individual must establish a cutoff point so that everything below it will be considered random "noise" and everything above it will be considered a signal worthy of attention. It has been hypothesized that stress causes the cutoff point to be lowered, thus increasing the number of signals correctly identified, but also increasing the frequency of false positives (Welford, 1973, pp. 567-580).

Those stressful events requiring behavioral adjustment on the part of health care managers can increase blood pressure by the conditioned "fight or flight response" in which increases occur in metabolism, heart rate, blood pressure, breathing, hyperventilation, and muscle response. While the fight or flight syndrome is still an essential ingredient for survival, the stresses of contemporary organizational life create a heightened problem for those experiencing this situation. Those who are under constant stress and who employ the fight or flight response have a greater chance of developing chronic hypertension, anxiety, gastrointestinal disorders, ulcers, colitis, and coronary heart disease, which may force them to retire prematurely from active organizational life prior to fully actualizing their potential and career.

Stress can be thought of as the individual's internal reaction to an environmental event. The stress response is a nonspecific psychological and physical series of events triggered by disruption to an individual's level of equilibrium. If this response is triggered often over long periods of time, there is a likelihood that latent physical and psychological disease will occur. Wear and tear on the system may not only involve progressive damage to the system, but in extreme form may result in the actual breakdown and disintegration of the system. We have seen that each individual has his own level of stress tolerance; when this level is exceeded, he "breaks down" physically and/or psychologically. And further exposure to the stress may lead to disintegration and death (Rahe & Lind, 1971, pp. 19-24).

An essential lesson to be digested by the health care manager is that complex problems which ultimately create stress can be solved in parts. One essential part of the health service delivery problem is effective management of those who work to deliver the services. Current pressures are being exerted upon all health care managers for more health services at lower costs. Health professionals are often placed in management positions where they are being held responsible for how effective they personally manage their system and also held responsible for the efficiency of the system they are involved with. Health care managers have a common problem in need of resolution: They lack the specific management training and development so necessary for managing conflict and reducing dysfunctional stress, which often characterize health care organizations functioning at less than rational levels.

## IRRATIONAL ORGANIZATIONS

Health care organizations often create a climate in which stress is one of the underpinnings of such activities as managing time, decision making, leadership, communications, motivation, and planning. It appears that heightened competition within the organization is a planned management strategy to increase productivity, since "to the winner, go the spoils." This creates internal competitiveness since the manager who is excessively competitive against his own standards is more likely to have physiological difficulty. Oftentimes, an individual may turn his anger on himself, in which case we see individuals who become their own worst enemies by repeatedly getting into difficulties, accidents, or, in extreme instances, turning their anger inward. When competition is extrinsically perceived and practiced, a limited reward system manifests apparent and hidden systems of intergroup conflict (Appelbaum, 1975, pp. 13-16). Instead of instigating competitive situations, management should emphasize departmental contributions (Appelbaum, 1977, pp. 39-44).

One of the most common situations producing fear, stress, and anxiety for the health care manager is change, which usually means some disruption of the status quo and ongoing relationships. Even a change for the better is perceived as a loss in which something has to be given up for a new replacement or system. For example, when highly controlled organizations become more decentralized, when previously authoritarian managers are asked to become more democratic, when dependent employees are required to become more aggressive, not only do they lose support, gratification, and goals, but they also must cope with new requirements for which they may be unprepared or unsuited (Levinson, 1976, p. 49). This situation of loss and new demands forces the individual caught in the middle to adapt quickly. But these psychological demands affect the individual through physiological or mental exhaustion. As an example, from the moment an individual gets his primary promotion he is caught in the middle, since he will always be responsible for subordinates and accountable to superiors. This ambivalent situation creates anger within the individual occupying the key managerial position under fire. There appear to be few outlets for this emotion which are organizationally acceptable and, therefore, the repression of anger is an important factor in almost all emotional illness. To put it another way, when you overload the circuits you are likely to blow a fuse, and when you overload the body with emergency demands, something eventually has to give. Overload in most systems leads to breakdown, whether we are dealing with single biological cells or managers in organizations (Miller, 1960, p. 116).

The scarcity of resources (such as financial and time) in addition to the need to contain costs creates other problems for the health care manager, which can only begin to be resolved within an open, responsive organizational climate. Well-designed managerial systems and interventions are essential in revitalizing counterproductive and maladaptive organizations. The competitive time-oriented battleground of the health care institution must be neutralized, since this climate produces stress and permanent damage to the system. Organizational research has focused upon this dilemma and even animal research has found that when male rats were paired to combat each other, approximately 80 percent of the defeated ones ultimately died although their wounds were not severe enough to warrant death. The British psychoanalyst Elliott Jacques (1973) contends that a peak in the death rate between 35 and 40 is attributable to the shock which follows the realization that an individual's life and career are on a descending path. This often creates a period of depression that increases the individual's vulnerability to stress-induced illnesses. This critical age for the vibrant manager (mid-30's) is when the upwardly mobile health care administrator must confront the fact that his hopes and targets are incongruent with reality since internal pressures for achievement are so intense that the pain of defeat is devastating. The essence of the problem is that the manager is underutilized but qualified to contribute. At best, to continue to develop, the manager now must either change his job, stagnate and accept it, seek external interests, or change careers. These are pessimistic alternatives for the individual trying to cope with and balance his world, life and organizational bind (Appelbaum, 1977, pp. 39-44). This dilemma creates further stress for the individual caught in the middle. The creation of stress symptoms is certainly not a simple or unimportant issue. To be maintained in a situation of unbalance between level of work and capacity, with or without excessive financial reward, leads to a combination of an individual unconsciously working towards breakdown, and a stress-inducing opportunity to collude unconsciously with a manager (Jacques, 1973, p. 154). Managers face this stressor at the perceived peak of their careers.

## TYPE A BEHAVIOR

Over the last half century or so, several observers have noted that certain work-related behaviors typically involving unmitigated striving and job involvement characterize numerous coronary patients (Friedman, 1969). Sir William Osler's lectures on angina pectoris before the Royal College of Physicians of London in 1910 included some particularly colorful observations. Of the 268 angina cases he personally encountered, 231 were men (Osler, 1910, pp. 696-700). Osler argued from a broad psychological perspective that it is not the delicate neurotic person who is prone to angina, but the robust, the vigorous in mind and body, the keen and ambitious man, the indicator of whose engines is always at "full speed ahead" (Osler, 1910, p. 839).

During the past 20 years or so, cardiologists Meyer Friedman and Ray Rosenman and their colleagues, working along the lines suggested by Osler and others, have more systematically described and studied what they have termed the Type A or coronary-prone behavior pattern and contrasted it with the Type B, or less coronary-prone behavior pattern (Friedman & Rosenman, 1973). In its extreme manifestations, each behavior pattern is alleged to represent a tightly woven pattern of habits, goals, characteristic modes of striving and achievement motivation, and personality traits. Persons displaying the Type A behavior pattern are overtly competitive, aggressive or even hostile, exceedingly demanding of self and others, and chronically restless, impatient, and *time* conscious. These individuals seemingly are never truly content unless battling multiple deadlines, obstacles, and harassments. There never seem to be enough hours in the day for Type As to get everything done; their cluttered calendars often serve as painful reminders of their incessant, compulsive striving. According to Friedman (1969), the Type A behavior pattern refers to a characteristic action-emotion complex which is exhibited by those individuals who are engaged in a chronic struggle to obtain an unlimited number of poorly defined things from their environment in the shortest period of time and, if necessary, against the opposing efforts of other things or persons in this same environment.

The reward structures in business and industry often facilitate the rise of Type As to higher status positions. It is also true that the competitive zeal and hard-driving qualities of Type As need not necessarily translate into vocational success. The attainment of high socioeconomic status is not, in this regard, analogous to a simple foot race with the prize awarded to the fastest (Type As) (Jenkins, 1975).

As a group, Type A subjects show higher serum cholesterol, higher serum fat, and more diabetic-like traits or precursors; smoke more cigarettes; exercise less (because they can't find time to do so); are "overdriving" certain of their endocrine glands in a manner that can be expected to damage their coronary arteries; have a tendency to develop blood clots; and suffer more from high blood pressure than Type B subjects (Friedman & Rosenman, 1973, p. 200).

It is interesting to note at this point that various health providers such as physicians and psychiatrists have been studied by Friedman recently and were found to favor Type A orientations. This can be explained by the dual life both often live between their practice and their academic appointments where "publish or perish" is still a stressful reality of their occupation, leading to constant struggle.

If this type of struggle becomes chronic, a commensurate excess discharge (also chronic) of various hormones occurs. Most Type A subjects not only discharge more norepinephrine and epinephrine (the nerve hormones or catecholamines), but also "overdrive" their pituitary glands to secrete too much ACTH (a hormone that stimulates the adrenal glands to discharge cortisol and other hormones) and growth hormone. Further, most Type A subjects exhibit an excess of the pancreatic hormone insulin in their blood—a sign generally believed to indicate that something is seriously wrong with the disposition of fat and sugar in the body. As a result of these abnormal discharges of catecholamines from the nerve endings and of hormones from the pituitary, adrenal, and pancreatic glands, most Type A subjects exhibit the unhealthy physiological characteristics just mentioned. In a sense, Type A subjects too often are exposing their arteries to "high voltage" chemicals even during the "low voltage" periods of their daily living (Friedman & Rosenman, 1973, p. 202).

Despite the distinction between Type A and Type B persons, the A-B variables were not intended to represent a typology but rather the endpoints of a normal distribution. Many persons demonstrate mixed aspects of Type A behavior, perhaps depending to some extent on differential social learning experiences and specific situational contingencies. Type Bs often display Type A characteristics (Glass, 1977).

Type As are overly achievement oriented, a point examined in a research study of over 4,000 employed men and women (Shekelle, Schoenberger, & Stamler, 1976, pp. 381-394). Type As demonstrated higher educational attainment and occupational prestige. Thus hard-driving Type A individuals are somewhat more likely to attain higher levels of educational and vocational success (at least as typically defined in contemporary Western societies) than their Type B peers.

Type A behavior is as clinically significant as the classical risk factors, including blood pressure and smoking, and subjects classified as Type A are approximately twice as likely to develop coronary heart disease as those classified Type B. At the time of a final eight-and-one-half year follow-up report, 11.2 percent of the men initially judged as Type A had developed coronary heart disease in contrast to 5 percent of the men judged Type B. In addition, Type As have been found more likely to suffer recurrent infarction (Jenkins, Zyzanski, & Rosenman, 1976, pp. 342-347).

Another research study (Dembroski & MacDougall, 1978, pp. 23-33) reported that coronary patients displayed a greater preference for working alone under pressure. Type As are concerned with maintaining control over environmental stressors. The motivation of Type As to actually confront stress alone may also reflect this strong desire for control. In fact, however, such a preference for isolation while under duress may increase responsibility, pressure, and job demand. The researchers further reported that subjects who showed a preference for working alone under stress also demonstrated greater cardiovascular reactivity. These studies represent an important contribution while further underlining the need for additional research examining the interaction of behavior pattern and stressful events.

## TENSION AND TIME

When managers are working under stress, the quality of their work is often affected as well as their efficiency. They then attempt to compensate for the loss in quality by increasing energy, tension, and time investment. When tension is excessive, it affects the working efficiency of the manager and may become psychologically disabling. Tension and anxiety can result in a feeling of helplessness for the manager, when he is working at less than half his potential efficiency. Tensions become very expensive when excessive and actually thwart the efforts of the manager.

The individual's judgment is affected as well, which creates problems with regard to decision making since the individual is now operating at a different perception level. When health care executives are attempting to make decisions, they employ integration, which is the synthesis of many diverse facts, and try to focus upon an overall conceptual pattern. When they face emotional stress and this stress is above an acceptable tolerance level, the critical psychological balance is lost and many of their normally insightful thoughts become extremely fragmented, therefore affecting their performance. When their ideas begin fragmenting in an uncontrolled manner, feelings of personal security are threatened, which leads to defensive behavior. The stress of attempting to maintain a level of equilibrium forces these managers to utilize their emotional reserves and develop defensive attitudes which are not usually employed under the low stress situations in which they are much more efficient. Thus an abundance of tension and stress wastes valuable time. In addition, too much tension traps the individual into a state of preoccupation with issues that are insignificant. The forcing of attention and time to these concerns creates a vicious cycle that must be broken at an early point in time. The more that managers understand the complexity of the problems that they are held responsible for, the more they will understand how limited their individual resources are for solving these problems and understand the need for help from subordinates.

Some managers who are in positions of authority feel quite guilty about the authority that has been given to them since they actually do not feel they should be there in the first place. This guilt usually creates more emotional stress and tension. As the individual develops, he has learned to keep these emotions under control and he is taught that it is perfectly acceptable to feel these but not acceptable to act them out. When the individual demonstrates how aggressive or frustrated he feels, it usually brings about retaliation on the part of others affected by it.

Most anxieties at managerial levels are caused by an overly developed superego on the part of the executive, feelings of inadequacy, or those guilt feelings that are often stimulated by the temptation to use power in a position which the executive feels he does not deserve in the first place. The North American culture is one in which managers have been trained to suffer in silence and therefore, if no one comprehends that they are experiencing anxiety and tension, they can still present a facade of adequacy. Managers must learn to distinguish between those anxieties that are valid and those anxieties which appeal to emotional needs. One way of doing this is to use trusted peers and colleagues as sounding boards to find out whether or not some of the concerns are valid. This, however, necessitates the utilization of trust, which is not an integral part of the interpersonal climate in most organizations.

## HEALTH CARE STRUCTURES

The organizational structure of the typical general hospital differs substantially from the bureaucratic model of many other large-scale organizations. This difference results from the unusual relationship between the formal authority represented by the administrative hierarchy and the authority of knowledge possessed by health professionals in the hospital. The hospital would be a much less complex institution if it did fit the typical pyramid. However, this is not the case. Only those people who work for the hospital (i.e., have their salaries paid by the hospital) typically fit into the pyramid. The medical staff, consisting of those physicians and professionals who have been authorized by the governing board to admit and attend patients in the hospital, does not fit into the pyramid, since they are generally not paid by the hospital but by their patients, and most physicians relish the independent nature of this relationship. Thus the hospital's organizational pattern is literally a dual pyramid (Longest, 1976, pp. 8-9).

This complex pattern becomes evident when one considers that almost no one in the organization has only one immediate superior (a highly desirable attribute of bureaucratic organizations). In fact, employees such as nurses must take orders from their own head nurse, who is a member of the administrative hierarchy, from the medical chief of their respective service, and, in regard to patients, from every individual physician on the medical staff. It is not uncommon for these orders to be contradictory, since each group of participants interprets the means for meeting objectives in terms of its own value systems and requirements. The hospital is in fact a very complex social system with substantial conflicts among the participants—patients, physicians, trustees, administrative staff, and paramedical personnel (Longest, 1976, p. 10).

The conflict experienced within this network can be quite stressful for managers of health care systems. Perhaps no single organizational problem facing these organizations is more important than that of developing a more effective working relationship between the hospital medical staff and administration. It appears that an active management strategy and intervention is required to reverse these health care conflicts in order to accomplish effectiveness, efficiency, and satisfaction. This takes time but time is also so scarce that additional demand on it leads to additional stress.

In examining the management of stress or the management of any organizational activity, the concept of management is brought to the front as a process intended to achieve organizational goals while fulfilling the needs of its members. Drucker (1977) states that management is a task and a discipline. He further adds (p. 11):

> But management is also people. Every achievement of management is the achievement of a manager. Every failure is a failure of a manager. People manage rather than forces or facts. The vision, dedication and integrity of managers determine whether there is management or mismanagement.

The management of stress within the dynamic health care system actually must begin with an understanding of the dynamics and counterproductive effects of induced organizational stress. The pattern of upward mobility at any cost leads to neurotic systems often too far advanced to manage the unresolved conflicts. Understanding the factors and sources of managerial pressure is only the first step in stress reduction (Cooper & Marshall, 1976, pp. 11-28). The basic responsibility for maintaining organizational and individual health is based on the relationship between administrative and medical staff and must take into account the dynamics of stress.

---

**REFERENCES**

Adams, J. Improving stress management. *Social Change: Ideas and Applications,* NTL Institute, 1978, *8*(4) 1-11.

Albrecht, K. *Stress and the manager.* Englewood Cliffs, N.J.: Prentice-Hall, 1979.

Appelbaum, S.H. An experiential case study of organizational suboptimization and problem solving. *Akron Business and Economic Review,* Fall 1975, *6*(3), 13-16.

Appelbaum, S.H. The middle-manager: An examination of aspirations and pessimism. *The Personnel Administrator,* January 1977, *22*(1), 39-44.

Appelbaum, S.H. Managerial-organizational stress: Identification of factors and symptoms. *Health Care Management Review,* 1980, *5*(1), 7.

Cooper, C.L., & Marshall, J. Occupational sources of stress: A review of the literature to coronary heart disease and mental ill health. *Journal of Occupational Psychology,* 1976, *49,* 11-28.

Dembroski, T.M., & MacDougall, J.M. Stress effects on affiliation preferences among subjects possessing the type A coronary-prone behavior pattern. *Journal of Personality and Social Psychology,* 1978, *36,* 23-33.

Drucker, P.F. *An introductory view of management.* New York: Harper and Row, 1977.

Friedman, M. *Pathogenesis of coronary artery disease.* New York: McGraw-Hill Book Co., 1969.

Friedman, M., & Rosenman, R.H. *Type A behavior and your heart.* New York: Fawcett Crest, 1973.

Glass, D.C. *Behavior patterns, stress, and coronary disease.* Hillsdale, N.J.: Erlbaum, 1977.

Jacques, E. *Work, creativity and social justice.* New York: International Universities Press, 1973.

Jenkins, C.D. The coronary-prone personality. In W.D. Gentry & R.B. Williams (Eds.), *Psychological aspects of myocardial infarction and coronary care.* St. Louis, Mo.: C.V. Mosby Co., 1975.

Jenkins, C.D., Zyzanski, S.J., & Rosenman, R.H. Risk of new myocardial infarction in middle-aged men with manifest coronary heart disease. *Circulation,* 1976, *53,* 342-347.

Kiev, A., & Kohn, V. *Executive stress.* New York: AMACOM, 1979.

LaPatra, J.W. *Health care delivery systems.* Springfield, Ill.: Charles C. Thomas, 1975.

Levinson, H. *Psychological man.* Cambridge, Mass.: The Levinson Institute, 1976.

Longest, B.B., Jr. *Management practices for the health professional.* Reston, Va.: Reston Publishing, 1976.

Mechanic, D. *Public expectations and health care.* New York: Wiley, 1972.

Miller, J.G. Information input overload and psychopathology. *American Journal of Psychiatry,* 1960, *8,* 116.

Osler, W. The Lumleian lectures on angina pectoris. *Lancet,* 1910, *1,* 696-700, 839-844, 974-977.

Rahe, R.H., & Lind, E. Psychosocial factors and sudden cardiac death: A pilot study. *Journal of Psychosomatic Research,* January 1971, *15*(1), 19-24.

Rogers, C.R. "Interpersonal relationships: USA 2000." In Jong S. Jun & William D. Storm (Eds.), *Tomorrow's organizations: Challenges and strategies.* Glenview, Ill.: Scott, Foresman and Co., 1973, p. 122.

Shekelle, R.B., Schoenberger, J.A., & Stamler, J. Correlates of the JAS type A behavior pattern score. *Journal of Chronic Diseases,* 1976, *29,* 381-394.

Sigerist, H.E. *Medicine and human welfare.* New Haven, Conn.: Yale University Press, 1941.

Welford, A.T. Stress and performance. *Ergonomics,* September 1973, *16,* 567-580.

Williams, R.B. Physiological mechanisms underlying the association between psychosocial factors and coronary disease. In W.D. Gentry & R.B. Williams (Eds.), *Psychological aspects of myocardial infarction and coronary care.* St. Louis, Mo.: C.V. Mosby Co., 1975.

Wren, D.A. *The evolution of management thought.* New York: Ronald Press, 1972.

Yates, J.E. *Managing stress.* New York: AMACOM, 1979.

# Chapter 9

# Interviews with Executive Directors of Three Hospitals Examining How They Manage Time

Interviews were held with the following hospital executive directors to ascertain how they effectively manage their time: Mr. Paul A. Scholfield, The Graduate Hospital, Philadelphia, Pennsylvania; Dr. Harvey Barkun, Montreal General Hospital, Montreal, Quebec; and Mr. Stephen Herbert, Royal Victoria Hospital, Montreal, Quebec.

The following questions were presented to each hospital administrator to elicit the insights, philosophy, and methodology each employs in fulfilling the requirements of his position and in managing the constraints of time both personally and professionally:

1. How do you effectively manage your time in your position as executive director?
2. Comment on the critical need for managing time in health care institutions as contrasted with corporations.
3. What pressures and/or stresses do you experience in managing your own time as chief executive officer of your hospital?
4. What are the time traps you experience?
5. Are you a juggler or a planner as administrator?
6. Do you manage scientifically by utilizing structure and strategic planning or do you find managing is an art?
7. What is your concept of delegation and the setting of priorities?
8. How do you insulate yourself from time interrupters when quiet time and planning are needed?
9. How do you measure your effectiveness in managing your role as executive director and managing your time?
10. What is your personal concept of time?

## Question No. 1:  How do you effectively manage your time in your position as executive director?

*Mr. Scholfield:*

The management of time is essentially the management of priorities. In order to establish priorities it is most essential to have your long-range plans developed and constantly in a condition of management awareness, so that your major objectives are always accomplished. The maintenance of priorities is done on a daily basis by working from a five-year long-range plan to a one-year set of specific goals and objectives as established institutionally through an MBO program and done on a daily basis through the hospital organizational structure and the executive director's daily and weekly schedule. I utilize a "day-timer organized activity," a mechanism whereby my administrative assistant writes for me twice daily, (A.M. and P.M.) an update for priority items which must get finished, i.e., meetings on the schedule, high-priority items for signature letters or reports that must be written, and decisions that must be made in that one half-day segment. Those segments are reviewed at the start of the half-day period by myself and the administrative assistant, and agreed to in terms of the priorities; then the priority items are always done in that half-day segment.

*Dr. Barkun:*

The basis for effectiveness really is the agenda that I lay down daily and spend a lot of time on. For instance, in meetings in my job I use this since a certain number of routine meetings are on a weekly basis, monthly basis, biweekly, and so on. At that point, I try as much as possible to have people who want to discuss a problem or want to discuss anything at all, make an appointment to see me so that I can plan my time in a better fashion. The only problem is that in a hospital you are constantly putting out fires and dealing with crises and I think it is even more true when you are a physician-administrator; I handle a number of problems like one I am involved with now which would normally be handled and fall to the director of professional services in Quebec or a medical director in the United States. Many of these problems go to a medical director, but unfortunately mine is away on a prolonged illness, and even when he is here, I handle a fair number of these problems myself. Therefore this adds to the load, you might say, in that medical problems which are perhaps only administrative spin-offs are coming into this office as well as purely administrative problems. So the management really is trying to set up an appointment system as much as possible, but then I always try and leave enough time free to put those fires out during the day.

The second aspect to be considered, I think, is the aspect of time spent outside the hospital, which involves government meetings, regional council meetings, and McGill University meetings, since I wear a second hat as Associate Dean at the

Faculty of Medicine, which takes a fair amount of my time. I always try to balance the two; the outside and the inside, since trying to delegate to good people inside is essential because a number of things done outside can only be done by me.

*Mr. Herbert:*

By screening, through secretarial staff, material coming in and the phone calls coming in. Also, by delegating wherever appropriate or possible and by not getting involved in those things that do not require my input or decision.

## Question No. 2: Comment on the critical need for managing time in health care institutions as contrasted with corporations.

*Mr. Scholfield:*

A health care institution is a community institution responsible for providing services to a large segment of the population/community at various levels. In addition the hospital administration has no direct control of its revenue sources; the revenue for the institution is done through the provision of services. All of the services are based on physician demand. Physicians schedule outpatient encounters, schedule outpatient services, admit patients, prescribe the diagnostic and therapeutic care required for the patients, prescribe surgery, perform the surgery, do the rehabilitative care within the confines of the institution, discharge patients, and prescribe home care or any follow-up care required. The administration responds to physician demand for services and provides those services, thereby generating institutional revenue. Whereas a corporation in either the product or service business has a marketing force and generates its own revenue through its own corporate structure. This difference requires the administration of a hospital to be responsive to its medical staff. The medical staff of a 300-bed hospital consists of approximately 100 active admitting physicians and 200 additional physicians at lesser levels of activity. A teaching hospital has the further complication of requirement of time interfaced with, in our case, the University of Pennsylvania, and all of the involvement in academic affairs, as well as all the time demands of the entire corporate structure.

*Dr. Barkun:*

Health care institutions have complexity. They have a major difference, I think, with normal industry or any marketing area, unless you have what I call a "parallel government structure" in which you have the administration and the medical staff. I am referring to hospitals or other health care structures which do not necessarily involve physicians, but at the Montreal General you do. The North American model has these two structures: an administrative government and a medical staff government, and the two come together at the medical director, executive director, and board levels. I therefore spend a lot of time dealing with communications between the medical staff and the administration. It makes for less of a line-type of operation which you may have in normal industry, where everything flows from the top down, orders are given, and decisions are taken. There is far more consultation and communication in the health care field, and what that does is it multiplies the number of meetings you need to have, and multiplies the number of people you have to see; you just don't pick up the telephone and have a meeting or just give an order. Much of it is done through consultation and some participation and that certainly adds to the complexity.

*Mr. Herbert:*

I am not sure that one can separate health care facilities or programs from other public sector programs or, in fact, industry. I think the only reasons one could say that this area is perhaps more intense in terms of need at this time is that there is a need to review all aspects of our operation to determine whether, in fact, activities are essential, and to ensure, where they are essential, that this is the most cost-effective way of conducting the operation. Because of limited financial resources there is also a need to carefully review and maintain momentum in the area of developments and techniques and ensure that a thorough analysis and evaluation is conducted on their viability and efficiency. Time must be used judiciously in order to be able to review and study.

**Question No. 3:  What pressures and/or stresses do you experience in managing your own time as chief executive officer of your hospital?**

*Mr. Scholfield:*

One of the realities is that there is not enough time to meet all of the demands that are placed on you as a director of a hospital—a major urban hospital and a teaching hospital. If you respond to the requirements I mentioned above and perform and represent the hospital in the health systems agency, in the local hospital council, and at the State and Federal levels, you have to appear to be accessible constantly to all of the demands placed on you. Going back to the revenue side of the equation, you are particularly vulnerable to those demands for your time and involvement from physicians who dictate your revenue sources. The appearance of accessibility has to be maintained by organizational staff, in my case administrative assistant and secretarial staff and associate directors. The executive director's office, in effect, responds to requests for time and only those that really require my involvement get directly to me. The greatest single pressure is simply not having enough time to go to all of the meetings and achieve all of the long-range objectives of the institution. It makes it difficult to be constantly responsive to an "open door policy" model and to demands made on your time.

*Dr. Barkun:*

I think the stresses are the same as everybody else's. There is the frustration of running overtime in meetings; there is the frustration of walking in at 8:00 or 8:30 A.M. and finding three people waiting for you that you didn't expect to see at all. What it does is more or less set your entire day off. There are emergency meetings constantly being called either in the hospital, at the University, by the Ministry, or by the Regional Council because of some crisis. I feel that in a business, if you wish, like ours, all you really have to give is your time and your knowledge. I feel very strongly that 80 percent of our business really is in communicating. I think that 80 percent of the problems arise through a lack of communication and that with proper communication you can solve them much more easily. Consequently, I have developed a little credo of my own. For instance, I put out about two memos a year—one says Merry Xmas, and the other says Happy New Year. I feel very strongly that if you put too many memos out they begin to lose their value, and they wind up in the "round file" rather quickly. Therefore, I think a memo isn't as good as a phone call, and by the same token I think a phone call is not as good as an "eyeball to eyeball" type of meeting. Therefore, I spend a lot of time walking the halls and talking to people and going to their office much more frequently than convening them to my office. All of which means time, especially when you've got an institution like this with 21 floors and a terrible elevator system which forces you to spend a lot of time on those elevators, going up and down. You try and keep fit by walking, but I walk down stairs, I don't walk up stairs. I think the priority lies with communication, and if that's going to force me to spend more time, I think it's worth it, because I think you get better communication by seeing people in person. But it does play havoc with your time management frame and consequently you find that at 6:15 in the evening there are a number of things which you wanted to do that have not been done. What that means is that I personally don't think I have ever missed coming in here on the weekend because that is my quiet time and when I can get off what Harvard would call an "in-basket exercise" to fulfill my commitments

*Mr. Herbert:*

Too many people want to see me, as well as the numerous involvements. At this time I have about eight people reporting directly to me in the organization, plus my activities with the Montreal Joint Hospital Institute, the Association of Hospitals of the Province of Quebec, the Regional Council, and a number of other associations and government or quasigovernment agencies. This requires time to think and any number of phone calls to interact or consult. These activities create certain pressures for an administrator.

## Question No. 4: What are the time traps you experience?

*Mr. Scholfield:*

There are time traps having to do with a back-up of paper work and a back-up of telephone calls. If you establish a pattern where you overschedule your day with meetings and you do not have sufficient time for paperwork or telephone calls, you will get backed up in one or another of those traps. If you constantly answer the phone as soon as the calls come in, you're basically on the phone approximately every three minutes and you do not have sufficient time to devote to priority report writing or reading. The other time trap that you get into is the trap of meeting schedules themselves in terms of the priority of demands: board level demands, physician demands, administrative demands, demands external to the institution, community-type demands, et cetera. So it is really a jockeying game in terms of keeping some scheduled meetings, a sufficiency of scheduled meetings to accomplish all of the priorities of the organization and your goals for the week, as well as your annual objectives. Administrators need sufficient flexibility to schedule meetings on a demand basis and then have the ability to do the paperwork and handle the telephone calls on a responsive basis.

*Dr. Barkun:*

I can give you examples of many of them where I leave the office and tell my secretary that I am going to see Dr. X, or Mr. Y, and I never get there, because I am buttonholed within ten yards of my office. Since the problem is of sufficient importance, we spend some time on it, and we either appear back in my office or go to the "buttonholer's" office. When I come back to the office and my secretary says, "I looked for you," I usually say, "Oh I forgot to go there afterwards." I hate to admit this, because I am supposed to be an executive who knows how to manage his time, but that's a trap! That's a terrible trap! It's a trap where you're in the middle, in the hub geographically in the hospital and you can be "attacked" or approached at almost any inopportune time. I used to have an open door policy, but I stopped that because you find people abuse it. You also find that people abuse your time by bringing problems to you (1) which should have been dealt with elsewhere or (2) that require spending far too much time with something that's not worth it. Those are traps, and you can't turn them off. You must deal with them.

*Mr. Herbert:*

Small crises such as getting involved in decisions where other people do not take the initiative or are reluctant; others involve government and outside agencies. Usually many of these can be dealt with by others in the organization but they end up on my desk. I think the very location of my office on the main floor contributes to the time traps; the boardroom is part of my suite and is used for meetings constantly. My accessibility ensures physicians that their needs and problems are directed to the most appropriate individual and/or mechanism in the organization to attend to their perceived requirements. This is my type of delegation.

## Question No. 5: Are you a juggler or a planner as administrator?

*Mr. Scholfield:*

I am a combination of both. The maximization or the efficient use of time is really effectively completing your priorities. Priorities have to be planned on an annual basis. Those plans have to be adjusted and, in my particular case, I do so via a regular monthly review of the annual objectives. The specific schedules and events to accomplish those are reworked weekly and, in my case, even twice a day. The twice-a-day activity turns out to be a juggling to reach an accommodation of the specific weekly and monthly plans. The chief executive officer of this organization, as well as any other corporate organization, has to respond in terms of crisis intervention; intervention because of a malpractice incident, intervention because of a demand by the media, or because of a death-and-dying situation—which occurs with much greater frequency in a hospital environment. The juggling is key because if you have only the ability to plan your work and work your plan, and respond rigidly, you become literally inaccessible. Inaccessibility is a cardinal sin for an administrator.

*Dr. Barkun:*

I am a juggler. I think we all plan, but then you have to juggle. You have to do both in a health institution. Like in any institution of any importance, you can't plan and just stick to your plan and not juggle from time to time. I think that is why I walk out into the hall as often as I do. I also think that is why I go to someone else's office, because I know very well I am going to run into ten people on the way to the office, but you do not get the "feel" of this kind of an institution unless you do things like that. When I was a medical director, just doing the medical administration, I used to spend at least 20 minutes every morning in the surgeon's room. I stopped doing surgery in 1959, but I still went to the surgeon's room and that is where you had a feel for how the "cutters" saw the world, and then you went down to emergency to see how they saw the world. You have to do things like that or else you are really insulated. But I wouldn't leave my door open to find out what is going on because of the abuse I got. People will abuse it . . . they stick their head in and I may be on a very important telephone call and they will still walk right in. But once you start to close your door, they don't do that anymore.

*Mr. Herbert:*

Some of both. Because of the state of the organization when I got involved, it was necessary to get very much into problem solving and a lot of juggling until new people came into the organization. In improving the foundation of the organization—of the operation, not physical—it became evident that the new directors that were being brought on could, with support, clearly initiate a planning process and, in dialogue, lay out plans to ameliorate some of the crises via some intervention. While I try to make as much time as possible available for planning, most of it usually occurs on weekends and evenings.

**Question No. 6: Do you manage scientifically by utilizing structure and strategic planning or do you find managing is an art?**

*Mr. Scholfield:*

I do part of both. The scientific, in terms of the quantitative assessment in our particular institution, is implemented through quantitative controls of the operation which are written into the organizational objectives, and through the MBO given to each of the associate directors and each of the department heads, so all individuals perform against certain quantitative objectives. These have to do with productivity performance, quality performance, specific attainment of objectives, managing within the constraints of the hospital operational budget, and quantitative assessment against variances to budget. In terms of the scientific approach, in behavioral terms we use a matrix type of management structure where many task forces are assembled and disassembled on an organization-wide basis, or project-by-project, with several ad hoc task forces appearing simultaneously such as those necessary to change an operating system. We also use systems which are necessary to space programming, those necessary to start up operation of a new hospital or new segments of a hospital, those necessary to get a planning agency application together, et cetera. The art of management really comes in the people-handling aspect, in terms of taking those things that you have as desired results and utilizing the strengths and weaknesses of all members of the organizational structure to accomplish those objectives. The art of managing people, managing your time, managing your own priorities, really comes from experience rather than from application of a strict scientific methodology.

*Dr. Barkun:*

Managing is like medicine. It is an art and a science. I think the people part of managing is more of an art, and the ''thing'' managing is far more of a science. A balance sheet is a balance sheet. How to get people to stay within budget is more of an art than a science. Sure, we have programs in cost controls, and I'll use that as an example, if you wish. That is when both come into play—the art and the science. One is the art of getting people to cooperate and look at their structure and look at their operation and be aware of cost constraints. The other is almost the pure science of mathematics, of dealing with a balance sheet and budget and all the rest that it entails. I probably place more emphasis on the art than the science.

*Mr. Herbert:*

No question but it's both. Strategic planning is essential in this era, especially with the politics and the need to devise clear strategies to cope with the operations. But I think that human interaction and motivating people—while some people have written on ways to go about it—has a large element of ''art.''

## Question No. 7:  What is your concept of delegation and the setting of priorities?

*Mr. Scholfield:*

The establishing of priorities is done for the organization at the senior level, chief executive officer level, of the organization, in conjunction with the board of directors. The board of directors, acting with and through the executive director, establishes programmatic priorities and endorses long-range program development priorities. The executive director, as head of the administrative organization, is charged with the responsibility for carrying out these priorities, as well as continuously updating them. In this organization, as in any other organization, the tasks have to be delegated to the various organizational levels. A hospital is very much a horizontal organization with a multiplicity of departments of unique character, so that delegation is absolutely essential. In our particular organizational structure, through the process of management objectives and in conjunction with quantitative controls, department heads and associate directors are given objectives to perform, resources to achieve those objectives with, and time constraints within which to work. The priorities that are established on a centralized basis must be attained. These managers have a great deal of flexibility through the authority which is given to them through the delegation process to define which objectives are met at which particular points of time in terms of daily, weekly, and monthly allocation of resources. The centralized quantitative checks in terms of management reports serve to review the specific associate director and department head successes in the achievement of priorities and allocation of responsibilities. I do not believe you can fully delegate without giving each of the levels of management some flexibility within the overall objectives of reestablishing priorities. You have to realize that each of these operational departments has very stringent demands, operational service demands, placed on them, which must be satisfied on a daily basis, and such service is in fact the revenue of the institution and therefore takes precedence, so they have to all have capability to plan as well as to juggle.

*Dr. Barkun:*

You set priorities as much as you can. I think priority setting has been highly oversold, just like I think planning has been highly oversold. I think the change aspect of institutions, and especially the Province of Quebec, is where I think we are going faster than anyone else in certain terms of health care institutions. The change is such that I get into great arguments with some members of my staff about long-term planning. I do not think you can do much long-term planning. I have done so much long-term planning which has gone to naught and which never came to anything, because of changes from outside the system which influence the strategy. My first meeting this morning at 9:30 was with someone who claimed he had a priority which was valid in 1971. Today, he is wondering why things haven't gone the way they should have. Well, priorities change from 1971 to 1980, so I think it is important when you're making firm decisions in terms of where your dollar is going to go and where your resources are going to be put for the next year or so. Certainly in terms of budget you have got to leave out priorities. If not, you never get anywhere. I deal with delegation, in terms of priorities, since I feel very strongly about delegation. I think there are a certain number of the American presidents that I respect, not because of what they did, but because of the people to whom they delegated authority and responsibility and the way they were recruited. I believe strongly in delegation since I feel everyone does certain things very well. I think I do certain things very well, but I do other things not as well. Those things which are delegated, I think, are delegated to people we have been able to recruit, who do those things extremely well. There is an old story which I like to repeat: We had a dean at McGill who was away a great deal, and somebody once asked him: "Who does all the work when you are away?" He responded: "The same people who do it when I'm here." And that's delegation! In this place you have to know medical, nursing, finance, plant, construction, unionism. You can't do it all. You must delegate. It's not a single operation type of process.

*Mr. Herbert:*

I would like to start in terms of addressing objectives. We have clear mission statements which are necessary before we set about finding the objectives, both in terms of direction for the 80s as well as institutional objectives to work toward the achievement of the institutional goals. While one can delegate the specific activities related to the attainment of certain goals, I think in this operation we tend to do it by the senior directors getting together to discuss directions and goals; this involves a process of consensus at the senior level of the organization which creates an opportunity for all senior members of the medical staff and all management staff to review, comment, critique, and make additions. The objectives are assigned to people, monitored, and discussed in terms of other priorities.

### Question No. 8:  How do you insulate yourself from time interrupters when quiet time and planning time are needed?

*Mr. Scholfield:*

You employ several tactics. Essentially, I have two tiers of secretaries for myself. I have a secretary who handles all incoming communication, whether that communication be letters, interoffice memos, telephone calls, or initial requests by people walking into the office demanding to see me. She opens all of the mail and initially handles all of the phone calls, but to the extent that any of the mail, people, or telephone calls must go elsewhere in the organization, she is the first level for screening. Those items that she is either completely or partially convinced would require my involvement or the involvement of my administrative assistant, she then forwards to my administrative assistant. A system is established for prioritizing the mail and memos into signatures required, absolutely high priority within the half-day time period, routine, daily, specialized reading, general reading, and reading for circulation purposes only. The telephone calls and the personal encounters are screened by my administrative assistant to determine whether it is appropriate to (a) make an adjustment in my schedule or (b) interrupt my meeting for the visitor and/or the phone call. Periods during the day are established for response to telephone calls, review with the administrative assistant for readjusting the meeting schedule, and determination of private interruptions. I do take telephone calls in the midst of meetings only if required.

*Dr. Barkun:*

I recruited a good administrative assistant, who is a great protector and who sometimes overperforms this activity. I know other secretaries who you just cannot get to let you see their boss. Sometimes they really turn you off, and their boss frequently doesn't know it. The number one way to insulate is by your secretary-receptionist, assistant, or however you want to phrase it—that's one way of doing it. The other way of doing it is from time to time to let people know you are not pleased with their interruptions. I go to lunch in the dining room, not because the food is good, but because you can get more ''scuttle-butt'' talk and get a feeling for the institution. On a minor detail I don't mind being stopped, but I get very upset when somebody sits down and says, "Look I want to discuss my problem." To me, that is a time interrupter because my lunch hour is only about 40 minutes long, and I like to change my act and thought processes during that time. And from time to time, maybe twice a year, I blast off at that person publicly and say, "Look you want to discuss a problem, I have an office, and I have a locale and that's what I'm there for, not now!" Word gets around quickly.

*Mr. Herbert:*

I am not sure that I do. Obviously some of these can be screened and dealt with before they get to me, either through the secretarial staff, or by scheduling meetings with sufficient frequency that the crisis intervention or the interruptions need not occur as regularly as they might otherwise. I think as Henry Mintzberg describes in *The Nature of Managerial Work,* you can start an activity but if there is a crisis one has to interact and get involved. I think as organizational procedures become more clearly established, many of the things that are clearly visible can be picked up by others in the organization. While that does not eliminate the problem, it reduces some of the crises.

## Question No. 9:  How do you measure your effectiveness in managing your role as executive director and managing your time?

*Mr. Scholfield:*

One measure of effectiveness is completion of the major institutional objectives in accordance with the time schedule. In the case of our institution we were in a management crisis/survival situation with some very specific objectives to be accomplished each of the first five years of my administrative involvement, in order to guarantee institutional survival. The overall effectiveness is the measurement of attaining those objectives. Specifically, we measure from the point of taking an institution operating at a major deficit and turning it around into a profitable operation, from getting a replacement building program approved by the planning agencies as we did, for getting such an institution financed, built ahead of schedule, below budget, continue the operational control of the institution so that fiscal integrity is maintained, implement successful marketing objectives to increase the size of the medical staff threefold, make major medical programmatic changes, and replace most of the major chiefs of service. Therefore, performance objectives are measured on an annualized basis, in terms of attaining the specific operational objectives of the institution on a smaller unit or daily basis. I think one of the basic measurements is to be able to finish the day and ascertain that most of the activities necessary to be completed in that given day were in fact completed, i.e., the meetings that had to be held were held; additional meetings that had to be scheduled were scheduled and successfully conducted; telephone calls were handled; paperwork was handled in a routine fashion, and the "candy store" was looked after. Also, the cash was balanced daily and the institution operated for that particular period at a profit. I think it's necessary to reevaluate on a time/increment basis (I use weekly and monthly) the success and measure of those periods of daily effectiveness. It is also absolutely essential that when all appears to go wrong and the daily schedules are blown, for whatever reasons, most specifically due to unpredictable types of demands on my time and/or the organization, we can catch up activities within the increment of a week or so as to not totally dilute the schedule.

### Dr. Barkun:

Well, I don't know if I ever know how effective I am at managing my time, unless I set certain priorities. You must set yourself some goals and you must be able to carry them out in a certain frame. But how effective are you? I feel, that is on the basis of your own satisfaction, whether you can keep your job or not determines if you are number one. I feel feedback from your own people and feedback from your associates, or those who work for you, and those you work for, is important in how you judge it. When the Minister of Health says nice things about the Montreal General, which he's done publicly, you know you've done a fairly decent job, as well as when people pay a compliment. People pay you compliments for many reasons and unfortunately sometimes it's not for the reason you think. But, that is not the case here.

### Mr. Herbert:

I guess the answer is in relation to objectives. I will choose one example: The hospital had its operating budget cut by $5.1 million and we were visited by two assistant deputy ministers to clearly point out the need to have a balanced budget. They required that we devise what they called a Financial Recovery Plan to clearly indicate how and within what time frame this would be achieved. One way to do this is just monitoring the attainment of the specific actions laid down in relation to this plan in order to ensure that we were on track, and in order to ensure that we do meet the objective agreed upon.

## Question No. 10: What is your personal concept of time?

### Mr. Scholfield:

Time is one of the most precious commodities that an administrator or an executive officer has under his control. Time is a resource in terms of mantime— personal and organizational mantime, to be utilized to accomplish and attain organizational objectives. Time is a constraint and time is also a factor to be invested. The management of time in terms of the establishment of personal and organizational priorities and the successful achievement of those personal and professional priorities, through the utilization of other people, is the art of management.

*Dr. Barkun:*

Time is a resource. Time is, as I said before, something that everybody has. It has greater or lesser importance for some people. To me, it's of extreme importance. I get very upset, for instance, when I feel I'm wasting time, and that occurs frequently. I had a colleague telling me the other day that he doesn't go to the swimming club any more because it takes him too much time to go downtown and get undressed, get into the pool, get dressed and go home. I can well understand that. I think that I would feel the same way. I, as much as possible, try and do two things at the same time, because I feel that strongly. Unfortunately, I understand that only Napoleon was able to do that. It's a resource and I think it's one of our most important resources. You can either make good use of it or you can make poor use of it. Time is like money, it's like material, like manpower, it's the fourth dimension.

*Mr. Herbert:*

It is a resource. Probably one of the most important resources. Its availability allows action and thought, and I think its management is critical to being able to address and see an organization progress.

# Index

## A

ABC analysis, 51-53
Academy for Contemporary Problems, 4
Accomplishment and hours, 1, 8
Achievement, 113
Achievement motivation, 25
ACTH, 230
Activities
  brevity of, 161
  combining of, 56
  control of, 25
  as goals, 23
  and objectives, 183
  sequencing of, 56-57
  volume of, 23
Activity orientation, 19, 20, 23, 27, 38
Activity trap, 19, 22-25, 27
Adaptation, 5, 175
Adaptive motivation, 26
Administering and authority, 142
Administrative colleague, defined, 154
Administrative subordinate, defined, 154
Agenda
  daily, 236
  for meetings, 34
  for telephone calls, 20, 32
Age and time, 5, 21
American Hospital Association, 105, 153

American Management Association (AMA), 225
Analysis, 93
  ABC, 51-53
  care, 68
  cost-benefit, 31
  cost-effectiveness, 97
  factor, 113
  functional, 147
  job, 10, 56
  personal time, 38
  self, 14-16, 54, 59
  systematic, 170
  techniques of, 41, 51-53
  value, 104, 131-136
Anger, repression of, 228
Anticipatory management, 5
Anxiety, 12, 19, 39, 42, 63, 219, 220, 221, 227, 231, 232
  and perception, 63-65
Apathy, 12
Appraisal, 104, 199
Arousal and performance, 226
Assessment activities, 42
Assigning vs. delegation, 58
Attitudes, 10
Authority, 59, 141, 194, 219
  and administering, 142
  decision-making, 59
  defined, 142
  and responsibility, 48

249

Patient care, 110
Pay
  and performance, 183
  and productivity, 187
PDO. *See* Personal development
  objectives
Pecuniary motivation, 26
People costs, 112
People-handling aspects of
  management, 242
Perception
  and anxiety, 63-65
  of time, 3, 21, 44
Performance, 67, 104, 175, 176, 189, 195
  and arousal, 226
  criteria for, 196
  and delegation, 42
  and effort, 183
  group, 196
  and MBO, 183-184
  measurement of, 187, 191
  and pay, 183
  reviews of, 198
  and rewards, 195
  standards of, 115, 191
Personal characteristics, 8
Personal development objectives
  (PDOs), 215-218
Personal enhancement, 113
Personal goals, 191, 195, 197
Personal interaction, 113
Personality of manager, 66, 140, 163
Personal time analysis, 38
Perspective, law of, 11
PERT. *See* Program Evaluation and
  Review Technique
Physical stress, 12
Physician productivity, 103, 104,
  107, 126-131
Physiological exhaustion, 228
Planning, 1, 6, 11, 16, 23, 38, 42,
  59, 63, 75, 79, 83, 85, 96, 100,
  104, 113, 114, 115, 122-123, 146,
  180, 182, 185, 241-242, 244
  of day's activities, 7
  formal, 1, 6, 175

foundation for, 190
  long-range, 100, 103, 114, 141, 236
  rational, 184-187
  strategic, 61, 76, 98-101, 243
  tactical, 98, 99
Planning, programming and budgeting
  system (PPBS), 76, 97-98
PM type supervision, 112
Political manager, 140, 163
POSDCORB, 146
Power blackout, New York City, 76
PPBS. *See* Planning, programming
  and budgeting system
*Practice of Management, The*, 176, 181
Preoccupation with time, 21
"Prerecorded" hidden agendas. *See*
  "Programmed tapes"
Present orientation, 192
Primary care teams, 61
*Principles of Scientific Management,
  The*, 146
Priorities, 7, 13, 15, 16, 31, 35, 57,
  58, 236, 241, 243-245, 247
  need for, 77-79
Probabilistic systems, 76, 95-96
Problems
  causes of, 27
  formulation of, 92-93
  solving of. *See* Problem solving
Problem solving, 27, 77, 79, 180,
  206-215
  Bennett's paradigm of, 94-95
  elements of, 94
  intuitive, 42, 64
Processing, 107
Process-maintenance oriented
  supervision. *See* Type M supervision
Procrastination, 19, 21, 35, 77
Productive time vs. elapsed time, 10
Productivity, 7, 16, 41, 105-111, 115,
  183
  and behavioral dimensions, 113
  and busyness, 1, 9, 19, 23
  defined, 103, 105
  and delegation, 60-62
  and hours, 25

# About the Authors

STEVEN H. APPELBAUM is currently Acting Chairman and Associate Professor of Management, Faculty of Commerce and Administration, Concordia University, Montreal, Quebec, Canada. He earned the Ph.D. from the University of Ottawa. He is a management consultant who has developed programs in management by objectives, organizational development, team building, and more for clients such as Union Carbide, Inc., the Graduate Hospital and Children's Hospital of Philadelphia, Rhone-Poulenc, Inc., and the Canadian College of Health Service Executives. He is the author of over 60 articles that have appeared in hospital, business, and health care journals and is a reviewer for *The Personnel Administrator*. Dr. Applebaum is an active member of the American Psychological Association, Academy of Management, and the American Hospital Association. He previously served as manager of personnel services for TRW, Inc., manager of organizational development for Union Carbide, Inc., and Assistant Professor of Behavioral Sciences at the graduate school of Pace University. Dr. Applebaum's most recent book is *Stress Management for Health Care Professionals*, published by Aspen Systems Corporation.

WALTER F. ROHRS, a former New York businessman, is a full-time faculty member of the Department of Economics and Business Administration at Wagner College, Staten Island, New York. He holds an M.B.A. from the Wharton Graduate School of the University of Pennsylvania, and a Ph.D. from the Graduate School of Business Administration of New York University. He has conducted many seminars in which concepts and techniques of management have been applied to the use of time in hospital administration. Recently, he prepared a training module in time management for the International Business Machines Corporation. Dr. Rohrs is a member of the Health Care Division of the Academy of Management.